T0214324

Lecture Notes in Computer Science 11827

More information about this series at http://www.springer.com/series/7412

Ninon Burgos · Ali Gooya ·
David Svoboda (Eds.)

Simulation and Synthesis
in Medical Imaging

4th International Workshop, SASHIMI 2019
Held in Conjunction with MICCAI 2019
Shenzhen, China, October 13, 2019
Proceedings

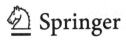 Springer

Editors
Ninon Burgos (iD)
Institut du Cerveau et de la Moelle
Épinière (ICM)
Paris, France

Ali Gooya (iD)
University of Leeds
Leeds, UK

David Svoboda (iD)
Masaryk University
Brno, Czech Republic

ISSN 0302-9743   ISSN 1611-3349   (electronic)
Lecture Notes in Computer Science
ISBN 978-3-030-32777-4   ISBN 978-3-030-32778-1   (eBook)
https://doi.org/10.1007/978-3-030-32778-1

LNCS Sublibrary: SL6 – Image Processing, Computer Vision, Pattern Recognition, and Graphics

This Springer imprint is published by the registered company Springer Nature Switzerland AG
The registered company address is: Gewerbestrasse 11, 6330 Cham, Switzerland

Preface

The Medical Image Computing and Computer Assisted Intervention (MICCAI) community needs data with known ground truth to develop, evaluate, and validate computerized image analytic tools, as well as to facilitate clinical training. Since synthetic data are ideally suited for this purpose, over the years, a full range of models underpinning image simulation and synthesis have been developed: (i) machine and deep learning methods based on generative models; (ii) simplified mathematical models to test segmentation, tracking, restoration, and registration algorithms; (iii) detailed mechanistic models (top–down), which incorporate priors on the geometry and physics of image acquisition and formation processes; and (iv) complex spatio-temporal computational models of anatomical variability, organ physiology, and morphological changes in tissues or disease progression.

The goal of the Simulation and Synthesis in Medical Imaging (SASHIMI)[1] workshop is to bring together all those interested in such problems in order to engage in invigorating research, discuss current approaches, and stimulate new ideas and scientific directions in this field. The objectives were to (a) hear from invited speakers in the areas of transfer learning, generative adversarial networks, variational auto encoders, and biophysical models to cross-fertilize these fields; (b) bring together experts of image synthesis to raise the state of the art; and (c) identify challenges and opportunities for further research. We also wanted to identify the suitable approaches to evaluate the plausibility of synthetic data and to collect benchmark data that could help with the development of future algorithms.

The 4th SASHIMI workshop was successfully held in conjunction with the 22nd International Conference on Medical Image Computing and Computer-Assisted Intervention (MICCAI 2019) as a satellite event in Shenzhen, China, on October 13, 2019. Submissions were solicited via a call for papers circulated by the MICCAI organizers, as well as by directly emailing colleagues and experts in the area. Each submission underwent a double-blind review by at least three members of the Program Committee, consisting of researchers actively contributing in the area. Compared to the 2018 edition, we saw an increased number of submissions and diversity of covered topics. At the conclusion of the review process, 16 papers were accepted. Overall, the contributions span the following broad categories in alignment with the initial call for papers: methods based on generative models or adversarial learning for MRI/CT/PET/microscopy image synthesis, image super resolution, and several applications of image synthesis and simulation for data augmentation, segmentation, or lesion detection. The accepted papers were presented within an oral session (5 papers) and a poster session (11 papers).

Finally, we would like to thank everyone who contributed to this fourth workshop: members of the Organizing Committee for their assistance; the authors for their

---

[1] http://www.sashimi.aramislab.fr.

contributions; the members of the Program Committee for their review work, promotion of the workshop, and general support; the invited speaker, Prof. Andreas Maier, for sharing his expertise and knowledge; the Steering Committee for their advice and support; and the MICCAI society for the general support.

October 2019

Ninon Burgos
Ali Gooya
David Svoboda

Organization

Organizing Committee

Ninon Burgos   CNRS - Brain and Spine Institute, France
Ali Gooya   University of Leeds, UK
David Svoboda   Masaryk University, Czech Republic

Steering Committee

Sotirios A. Tsaftaris   University of Edinburgh, UK
Alejandro F. Frangi   University of Sheffield, UK
Jerry L. Prince   Johns Hopkins University, USA

Program Committee

Navid Alemi Koohbanani   University of Warwick, UK
Ninon Burgos   CNRS - Brain and Spine Institute, France
Aaron Carass   The Johns Hopkins University, USA
Hamid Fehri   University of Oxford, UK
Ali Gooya   University of Leeds, UK
Matteo Maspero   UMC Utrecht, The Netherlands
Martin Maška   Masaryk University, Czech Republic
Jack Noble   Vanderbilt University, USA
Dzung Pham   Henry Jackson Foundation, USA
Nishant Ravikumar   University of Leeds, UK
Snehashis Roy   Henry Jackson Foundation, USA
David Svoboda   Masaryk University, Czech Republic
Vladimír Ulman   Max Planck Institute, Germany
Devrim Unay   Izmir University of Economics, Turkey
François Varray   Creatis, France
Arezoo Zakeri   University of Leeds, UK
Ting Zhao   Janelia Research Campus, USA

Contents

Empirical Bayesian Mixture Models for Medical Image Translation

Mikael Brudfors[1]([✉]), John Ashburner[1], Parashkev Nachev[2],
and Yaël Balbastre[1]

[1] Wellcome Centre for Human Neuroimaging, UCL, London, UK
{mikael.brudfors.15,j.ashburner,y.balbastre}@ucl.ac.uk
[2] UCL Institute of Neurology, London, UK
p.nachev@ucl.ac.uk

Abstract. Automatically generating one medical imaging modality from another is known as medical image translation, and has numerous interesting applications. This paper presents an interpretable generative modelling approach to medical image translation. By allowing a common model for group-wise normalisation and segmentation of brain scans to handle missing data, the model allows for predicting entirely missing modalities from one, or a few, MR contrasts. Furthermore, the model can be trained on a fairly small number of subjects. The proposed model is validated on three clinically relevant scenarios. Results appear promising and show that a principled, probabilistic model of the relationship between multi-channel signal intensities can be used to infer missing modalities – both MR contrasts and CT images.

1 Introduction

This paper concerns a relatively simple method of synthesising data of one medical image modality, from data of other modalities. This is known as 'image translation'. Applications of medical image translation are numerous, and include *e.g.* harmonising data across scanners; synthesising computed tomography (CT) images from magnetic resonance (MR) images for positron emission tomography (PET) attenuation correction [1], or decrease the need for radiating a patient; simplifying the problem of multi-modal image registration [2]; or generalising machine learning techniques by transferring out-of-distribution input data to the domain of the model's training data [3].

Mapping from the signal intensities of one modality to those of another can be loosely categorised as either optimisation- or learning-based. Optimisation-based methods rely only on the data at hand to optimise a mapping between modalities, and do not use training data. Examples include using non-parametric joint histograms [4], estimating an intensity transformation during image registration [5], and biophysical models [6]. Learning-based methods use training data to learn the mapping, and can be applied to translating an unseen image from one domain into another. Some examples in this category use clustering

N. Burgos et al. (Eds.): SASHIMI 2019, LNCS 11827, pp. 1–12, 2019.
https://doi.org/10.1007/978-3-030-32778-1_1

[7], random forests [8], patch-matching [9] and dictionaries [10]. Learning-based methods based on various convolutional neural network architectures are currently the most popular approach for this. Trained end-to-end, on either paired or unpaired training data [11–13], they show promising results at this task, although they can run the risk of hallucinating unwanted features [14].

This paper presents a more interpretable generative modelling approach to image translation. It could be classed as an optimisation-based approach, although it does use training data to learn priors that inform the optimisation of mappings. More specifically, we show how a generative model for group-wise normalisation and segmentation of neuroimaging data can be extended to handle missing data. The generative model has a Gaussian mixture model component, which can naturally handle missing data [15]. In this paper, we extend this missing data model to a variational Gaussian mixture. Fitting this model to various populations of medical images allows us to predict, from a few MR contrasts, entirely missing modalities (*e.g.*, non-acquired MR contrasts or CT images).

2   Methods

The prediction of one modality from another is here cast as a joint intensity modelling problem. The workhorse of the proposed method is the unified segmentation model [16], which uses mixtures of Gaussians with non-stationary tissue priors derived from a deformable template. When a large dataset is available, the optimisation of the template can be interleaved with the mixture model fit to each individual subject [17]. Furthermore, priors over the intensity parameters of the Gaussian mixture – its means and covariances – can be defined and optimised as well. This type of learning, where subject-specific parameters are marginalised while population parameters are optimised, is known as parametric empirical Bayesian methods [18]. Here, exact marginalisation is intractable, so we resort to a variational approximation.

Fully Observed Model: Let $\boldsymbol{X} \in \mathbb{R}^{D \times M}$ be a multimodal dataset from one subject, where M is the number of modalities and D is the number of voxels in the images. Each voxel is assumed to belong to one of K classes, where the classification is encoded by the label matrix $\boldsymbol{Z} \in [0, 1]^{D \times K}$, with $z_{dk} = 1$ *iff*. voxel d belongs to class k. Each tissue class is associated with a multivariate Gaussian distribution of dimension M, which encodes the intensities' mean ($\boldsymbol{\mu}_k \in \mathbb{R}^M$) and covariance ($\boldsymbol{\Sigma}_k \in \mathbb{R}^{M \times M}$) over the modalities. The Gaussian mixture model can then be written as a conditional probability that factorises across voxels:

$$p\left(\boldsymbol{X} \mid \boldsymbol{Z}, \boldsymbol{\mu}_{1\ldots K}, \boldsymbol{\Sigma}_{1\ldots K}\right) = \prod_{d=1}^{D} \prod_{k=1}^{K} \mathcal{N}\left(\boldsymbol{x}_d \mid \boldsymbol{\mu}_k, \boldsymbol{\Sigma}_k\right)^{z_{dk}}. \tag{1}$$

Subject-specific parameters (the label matrix and Gaussian parameters) are assumed to be drawn from prior distributions that describe their variability at the population level. Labels are drawn from a categorical distribution whose probabilities are encoded by a deformable template $\boldsymbol{a} \in \mathbb{R}^{D_a \times K}$. This template is mapped to the subject's brain using a non-linear deformation field $\boldsymbol{\phi}$. This assumption can be written as the conditional likelihood:

$$p(\boldsymbol{Z}) = \prod_{d=1}^{D} \text{Cat}(\boldsymbol{z}_d \mid \boldsymbol{\pi}_d), \quad \boldsymbol{\pi}_d \in \mathbb{R}^K, \quad \pi_{dk} = \frac{\exp(\omega_k + \boldsymbol{a}_{dk}(\boldsymbol{\phi}))}{\sum_{j=1}^{K} \exp(\omega_j + \boldsymbol{a}_{dj}(\boldsymbol{\phi}))}, \quad (2)$$

where $\boldsymbol{\omega} \in \mathbb{R}^K$ is a vector of global class proportions, which can be optimised to account for variable amounts of different classes (an example when modelling brain images could be atrophy due to ageing). The Gaussian parameters are drawn from their conjugate Gauss-Wishart distribution:

$$p\left(\boldsymbol{\mu}_k, \boldsymbol{\Sigma}_k^{-1}\right) = \mathcal{NW}\left(\boldsymbol{\mu}_k, \boldsymbol{\Sigma}_k^{-1} \mid \boldsymbol{\mu}_{0k}, b_{0k}, \boldsymbol{V}_{0k}, \nu_{0k}\right)$$
$$= \mathcal{N}\left(\boldsymbol{\mu}_k \mid \boldsymbol{\mu}_{0k}, \boldsymbol{\Sigma}_k/b_{0k}\right) \mathcal{W}\left(\boldsymbol{\Sigma}_k^{-1} \mid \boldsymbol{V}_{0k}, \nu_{0k}\right). \quad (3)$$

Assuming that all population parameters are fixed, a mean-field approximation is made so that the posterior distribution over all latent, subject-specific parameters factorises as:

$$q\left(\boldsymbol{Z}, \boldsymbol{\mu}_{1\ldots K}, \boldsymbol{\Sigma}_{1\ldots K}^{-1}\right) = \left[\prod_{d=1}^{D} q\left(\boldsymbol{z}_d\right)\right] \left[\prod_{k=1}^{K} q\left(\boldsymbol{\mu}_k, \boldsymbol{\Sigma}_k^{-1}\right)\right], \quad (4)$$

with $q(\boldsymbol{z}_d) = \text{Cat}(\boldsymbol{z}_d \mid \tilde{\boldsymbol{z}}_d)$ and $q\left(\boldsymbol{\mu}_k, \boldsymbol{\Sigma}_k^{-1}\right) = \mathcal{NW}\left(\boldsymbol{\mu}_k, \boldsymbol{\Sigma}_k^{-1} \mid \tilde{\boldsymbol{\mu}}_k, \tilde{b}_k, \tilde{\boldsymbol{V}}_k, \tilde{\nu}_k\right)$. The posterior parameters (denoted by a tilde) can be optimised in turn by maximising the evidence lower bound (ELBO):

$$\mathcal{L} = \mathbb{E}\left[\ln p\left(\boldsymbol{X} \mid \boldsymbol{Z}, \boldsymbol{\mu}_{1\ldots K}, \boldsymbol{\Sigma}_{1\ldots K}\right)\right]$$
$$- \sum_{d=1}^{D} \text{D}_{\text{KL}}\left(q_{\boldsymbol{z}_d} \parallel p_{\boldsymbol{z}_d}\right) - \sum_{k=1}^{K} \text{D}_{\text{KL}}\left(q_{\boldsymbol{\mu}_k, \boldsymbol{\Sigma}_k} \parallel p_{\boldsymbol{\mu}_k, \boldsymbol{\Sigma}_k}\right). \quad (5)$$

When multiple subjects $\{\boldsymbol{X}_n\}_{n=1}^{N}$ are processed, the posterior distribution factorises across subjects and a combined ELBO can be written by summing the individual ELBOs ($\mathcal{L} = \sum_{n=1}^{N} \mathcal{L}_n$). In this case, empirical population priors can be obtained by optimising the combined ELBO with respect to the template ($\boldsymbol{a}$) and Gauss-Wishart prior hyper-parameters ($\boldsymbol{\mu}_{0k}, b_{0k}, \boldsymbol{V}_{0k}, \nu_{0k}$). The means and scale matrices have closed form solutions, while the template and degrees of freedom must be optimised using an iterative scheme. Population prior parameters and subject posterior parameters can be optimised in turn, resulting in a variational Expectation-Maximisation (VEM) algorithm [19].

Missing Modalities: Let us assume that some modalities are missing in a voxel[1]. We write as $\boldsymbol{o}$ the vector indexing observed modalities and as $\boldsymbol{m}$ the

---

[1] For example, a multi-channel MRI might have three contrasts: T1w, T2w and PDw. In one voxel, only the T1w intensity is observed. The T2w and PDw intensities are then assumed missing in that voxel. Note that different voxels can have different combinations of contrasts/modalities missing.

vector indexing missing modalities. Therefore, the observed channels can be written as $g = x_o$ and the missing channels as $h = x_m$, where the voxel index d has been temporarily dropped for clarity. For a voxel in class k, the marginal distribution of the observed channels can then be written as [20]:

$$p\left(g \mid \mu_k, \Sigma_k, z_k = 1\right) = \mathcal{N}\left(g \mid \mu_{ko}, \Sigma_{koo}\right), \tag{6}$$

and the conditional distribution of the missing channels as:

$$
\begin{aligned}
&p\left(h \mid g, \mu_k, \Sigma_k, z_k = 1\right) = \\
&\mathcal{N}\left(h \mid \mu_{km} - \left(\Lambda_{kmm}\right)^{-1} \Lambda_{kmo}\left(g - \mu_{ko}\right), \left(\Lambda_{kmm}\right)^{-1}\right),
\end{aligned} \tag{7}
$$

where the precision matrix $\Lambda = \Sigma^{-1}$ is the inverse of the covariance matrix.

The set of all missing values in an image is written as $\mathcal{H} = \{h_d\}_{d=1}^D$. The mean field approximation becomes:

$$q\left(\mathcal{H}, Z, \mu_{1...K}, \Sigma_{1...K}^{-1}\right) = \left[\prod_{d=1}^D q\left(h_d \mid z_d\right) q\left(z_d\right)\right]\left[\prod_{k=1}^K q\left(\mu_k, \Sigma_k^{-1}\right)\right], \tag{8}$$

where $q\left(h_d \mid z_d\right) = \prod_{k=1}^K \mathcal{N}\left(h_d \mid \tilde{h}_{dk}, \tilde{S}_{dk}\right)^{z_{dk}}$. The marginal posterior over missing values is a mixture of Gaussians that can be obtained by marginalising the labels:

$$q(h_d) = \sum_{k=1}^K \tilde{z}_{dk}\mathcal{N}\left(h_d \mid \tilde{h}_{dk}, \tilde{S}_{dk}\right). \tag{9}$$

Its expected value is $\mathbb{E}\left[h_d\right] = \sum_k \tilde{z}_{dk}\tilde{h}_{dk}$. This is the expression that we evaluate to predict missing voxels.

The set of all observed values is written as $\mathcal{G} = \{g_d\}_{d=1}^D$. The ELBO can then be written in two equivalent forms:

$$
\begin{aligned}
\mathcal{L} =\ &\mathbb{E}\left[\ln p\left(\mathcal{G} \mid Z, \mu_{1...K}, \Sigma_{1...K}\right)\right] \\
&- \sum_{d=1}^D D_{\text{KL}}\left(q_{z_d} \parallel p_{z_d}\right) - \sum_{k=1}^K D_{\text{KL}}\left(q_{\mu_k, \Sigma_k} \parallel p_{\mu_k, \Sigma_k}\right)
\end{aligned} \tag{10}
$$

$$
\begin{aligned}
\mathcal{L} =\ &\mathbb{E}\left[\ln p\left(X \mid Z, \mu_{1...K}, \Sigma_{1...K}\right)\right] - \sum_{d=1}^D \mathbb{E}_{z_d}\left[D_{\text{KL}}\left(q_{h_d\mid z_d} \parallel p_{h_d\mid z_d}\right)\right] \\
&- \sum_{d=1}^D D_{\text{KL}}\left(q_{z_d} \parallel p_{z_d}\right) - \sum_{k=1}^K D_{\text{KL}}\left(q_{\mu_k, \Sigma_k} \parallel p_{\mu_k, \Sigma_k}\right).
\end{aligned} \tag{11}
$$

The first form is used to optimise the labels' posterior parameters, while the second is used to optimise, in turn, the missing values and the Gaussian posterior parameters.

Model Updates: Optimising the ELBOs in (10) and (11) gives the subject-level update equations as:

$$\tilde{z}_{dk} = \frac{\exp\left(\mathbb{E}\left[\ln \mathcal{N}\left(\boldsymbol{g}_d \mid \boldsymbol{\mu}_k, \boldsymbol{\Sigma}_k\right)\right] + \ln \pi_{dk}\right)}{\sum_{l=1}^{K} \exp\left(\mathbb{E}\left[\ln \mathcal{N}\left(\boldsymbol{g}_d \mid \boldsymbol{\mu}_l, \boldsymbol{\Sigma}_l\right)\right] + \ln \pi_{dl}\right)}. \tag{12}$$

$$\tilde{b}_k = b_{0k} + \sum_{d=1}^{D} \tilde{z}_{dk} \tag{13}$$

$$\tilde{\boldsymbol{\mu}}_k = \frac{b_{0k}\boldsymbol{\mu}_{0k} + \sum_{d=1}^{D} \mathbb{E}\left[z_{dk}\boldsymbol{x}_d\right]}{\tilde{b}_k} \tag{14}$$

$$\tilde{\nu}_k = \nu_{0k} + \sum_{d=1}^{D} \tilde{z}_{dk} \tag{15}$$

$$\tilde{\boldsymbol{V}}_k^{-1} = \nu_{0k}\boldsymbol{V}_{0k}^{-1} + \sum_{d=1}^{D} \mathbb{E}\left[z_{dk}\boldsymbol{x}_d\boldsymbol{x}_d^{\mathrm{T}}\right] + b_{k0}\boldsymbol{\mu}_{k0}\boldsymbol{\mu}_{k0}^{\mathrm{T}} - \tilde{b}_k\tilde{\boldsymbol{\mu}}_k\tilde{\boldsymbol{\mu}}_k^{\mathrm{T}} \tag{16}$$

The update equations for the Gaussian parameters in the missing data case are very similar to the fully observed case, except that expectations are taken about the data. These expectations are evaluated as:

$$\begin{aligned}
\mathbb{E}\left[z_{dk}\boldsymbol{x}_d\right]_o &= \tilde{z}_{dk}\boldsymbol{g}_d, & \mathbb{E}\left[z_{dk}\boldsymbol{x}_d\boldsymbol{x}_d^{\mathrm{T}}\right]_{mm} &= \tilde{z}_{dk}\left(\tilde{\boldsymbol{h}}_{dk}\tilde{\boldsymbol{h}}_{dk}^{\mathrm{T}} + \tilde{\boldsymbol{S}}_{dk}\right), \\
\mathbb{E}\left[z_{dk}\boldsymbol{x}_d\right]_m &= \tilde{z}_{dk}\tilde{\boldsymbol{h}}_{dk}, & \mathbb{E}\left[z_{dk}\boldsymbol{x}_d\boldsymbol{x}_d^{\mathrm{T}}\right]_{om} &= \tilde{z}_{dk}\boldsymbol{g}_d\tilde{\boldsymbol{h}}_{dk}^{\mathrm{T}}, \\
\mathbb{E}\left[z_{dk}\boldsymbol{x}_d\boldsymbol{x}_d^{\mathrm{T}}\right]_{oo} &= \tilde{z}_{dk}\boldsymbol{g}_d\boldsymbol{g}_d^{\mathrm{T}}, & \mathbb{E}\left[z_{dk}\boldsymbol{x}_d\boldsymbol{x}_d^{\mathrm{T}}\right]_{mo} &= \tilde{z}_{dk}\tilde{\boldsymbol{h}}_{dk}\boldsymbol{g}_d^{\mathrm{T}},
\end{aligned} \tag{17}$$

where

$$\tilde{\boldsymbol{h}}_{dk} = \tilde{\boldsymbol{\mu}}_{km} - \tilde{\boldsymbol{\Lambda}}_{kmm}^{-1}\tilde{\boldsymbol{\Lambda}}_{kmo}\left(\boldsymbol{g}_d - \tilde{\boldsymbol{\mu}}_{ko}\right), \qquad \tilde{\boldsymbol{S}}_{dk} = \tilde{\boldsymbol{\Lambda}}_{kmm}^{-1}, \tag{18}$$

and $\tilde{\boldsymbol{\Lambda}}_k = \tilde{\nu}_k\tilde{\boldsymbol{V}}_k$ is the posterior expected precision matrix of a given class.

Finally, we provide the optimal updates of the Gaussian prior parameters, given a set of individual posterior parameters. All prior parameters have closed-form updates, except for the degrees of freedom of the Wishart distribution, which is updated using an iterative Gauss-Newton scheme. The update equations are:

$$\boldsymbol{\mu}_{0k} = \left(\sum_{n=1}^{N} \tilde{\nu}_{nk}\tilde{\boldsymbol{V}}_{nk}\right)^{-1}\left(\sum_{n=1}^{N} \tilde{\nu}_{nk}\tilde{\boldsymbol{V}}_{nk}\tilde{\boldsymbol{\mu}}_{nk}\right), \tag{19}$$

$$b_{0k}^{-1} = \frac{1}{NM}\sum_{n=1}^{N} \tilde{\nu}_{nk}\left(\boldsymbol{\mu}_{0k} - \tilde{\boldsymbol{\mu}}_{nk}\right)^{\mathrm{T}}\tilde{\boldsymbol{V}}_{nk}\left(\boldsymbol{\mu}_{0k} - \tilde{\boldsymbol{\mu}}_{nk}\right), \tag{20}$$

$$\boldsymbol{V}_{0k} = \frac{1}{N\nu_{0k}}\sum_{n=1}^{N} \tilde{\nu}_{nk}\tilde{\boldsymbol{V}}_{nk}, \tag{21}$$

$$\frac{\partial \mathcal{L}}{\partial \nu_{0k}} = -\frac{1}{2} \left(N \left(\ln |\mathbf{V}_{0k}| + \psi_M \left(\frac{\nu_{0k}}{2} \right) \right) - \sum_{n=1}^{N} \left(\ln \left| \tilde{\mathbf{V}}_{nk} \right| - \psi_M \left(\frac{\tilde{\nu}_{nk}}{2} \right) \right) \right),$$

(22)

$$\frac{\partial^2 \mathcal{L}}{\partial \nu_{0k}^2} = -\frac{N}{4} \psi_M' \left(\frac{\tilde{\nu}_{0k}}{2} \right).$$

(23)

We do not provide update rules for the template ($\boldsymbol{a}$), as they can be found in [17].

3   Experiments and Results

In this section we aim to explore the translation (or inference) capability of the proposed model by conducting three experiments on publicly available data. We investigate: (1) inferring missing voxels of MRIs with differing field of views; (2) inferring entirely missing MRI contrasts; and (3), inferring CT scans from MRIs. The findings are quantified by computing the peak-signal-to-noise-ratio (PSNR) for an image channel c as:

$$\text{PSNR} = 10 \log_{10} \frac{maxval^2}{MSE},$$

(24)

where the mean-squared error is defined as MSE $= \frac{1}{D} \sum_{d=1}^{D} (\hat{x}_{cd} - (\mathbb{E}[\boldsymbol{h}_d])_c)^2$, $maxval$ is the maximum channel intensity in the reference image $\hat{\boldsymbol{X}}$, and $\mathbb{E}[\boldsymbol{h}_d]$ from (9) is evaluated to predict missing voxels. The PSNR is a metric that is commonly used in the medical image synthesis literature [11–13]. Note that no voxels are excluded when computing the PSNR.

3.1   MRI Contrast Translation

This section evaluates translating between MR contrasts. The model is trained on 50 subjects from the publicly available IXI dataset[2], which was acquired on three different MR scanners[3]. Each IXI subject has three MR images: a T1-, T2- and PD-weighted scan (T1w, T2w and PDw). Furthermore, the images have approximately 1 mm isotropic voxels and all subjects are healthy. $K = 12$ mixture components are used, resulting in the model shown in Fig. 1. Note that the template learned by the algorithm does not need to represent real tissues. Here, the model has been treated as a method of representing a probability density function, rather than as a way to do clustering. Any 'meaningful' clusters are incidental.

---

[2] http://brain-development.org/ixi-dataset/.

[3] This scenario is more realistic in a clinical context. The results would improve if data from only one scanners was used.

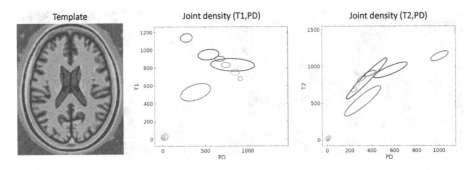

Fig. 1. Template and expectations of the Gaussians drawn from the Gauss-Wishart priors, learnt from 50 IXI subjects. Densities are plotted using their 3σ isocontours. This model is fit to a new subject, which allows for inferring missing voxels.

Inferring MRIs with Differing Fields of View: Doctors often acquire routine clinical MR scans of multiple contrasts. Commonly, these contrasts have differing fields of view, meaning the brain coverage varies (*cf.* observed T1w and T2w images in Fig. 2). This can be problematic for image segmentation routines as voxels with non-observed contrasts need to be discarded. The model should prevent this issue by inferring the values of these missing voxels. To test this, T1w, T2w and PDw scans of 50 unseen IXI subjects are used[4]. All of the voxels are retained in the PDw image, while an increasing amount of voxels are removed from the T1w and T2w images (25%, 50%, 75% and 100%). The missing voxels are then inferred with the trained model. An example can be seen in Fig. 2. The mean PSNR computed between the known references and the inferred images are shown in Table 1. For routine clinical MRI, it is rare that more than 50% of the field of view is missing. The results therefore suggest that the model does a good job at filling in missing fields of view, which could be of value in segmenting hospital data.

Inferring MR Contrasts: Could the proposed model be used to infer an entirely missing MR contrast? An interesting application for this type of MRI translation could be for segmentation methods based on deep learning. A deep learning model that has been trained on MR images of a specific contrast can overfit to its training data [21]. If images could be simulated as to match the training data of the deep learning model, it might generalise better.

To test how well the model predict a missing contrast the same IXI subjects as in the previous experiment are used. For each subject, all combinations of contrasts are permuted over, set as either observed or missing. For example, we observe just the T1w image and infer the T2w and PDw scans, or we observe the T2w and PDw scans and infer the T1w (see Fig. 3). The results from this experiment are shown in Table 2. These results imply that the T1w image is the most predictive, as the lowest PSNR is obtained when this contrast is missing.

---

[4] The model is trained on IXI subjects IXI[064--118], and tested on IXI[002--063].

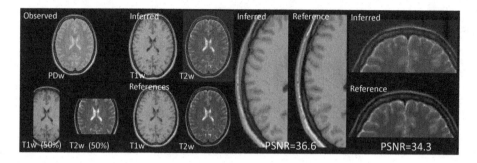

Fig. 2. Example of inferring MRIs with differing field of views. An MR image with three channels (PDw, T1w and T2w) is observed. The PDw scan has full brain coverage, while the T1w and T2w scans have partial brain coverage (50% of voxels removed in each channel). From the observed data the values of the missing T1w and T2w voxels are inferred. The reference T1w and T2w scans are shown for comparison, as well as PSNR values.

Table 1. Results for inferring MR images with different fields of view (for 50 subjects). The PSNR is computed between known T2w and PDw references and inferred images, where an increasing percentage of the field of view has been removed. Results are shown as mean ± std.

Contrast	PSNR			
	25%	50%	75%	100%
T1w	42.1 ± 1.6	36.3 ± 1.3	31.1 ± 1.3	28.9 ± 1.2
T2w	40.7 ± 2.1	34.4 ± 2.0	30.4 ± 1.8	27.6 ± 1.6

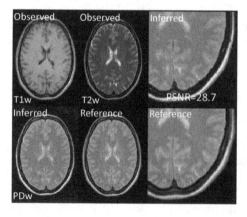

Fig. 3. Example of inferring non-acquired MR contrasts. An MR image with two channels (T1w and T2w) is observed. The PDw scan is missing, but inferred from the observed T1w and T2w scans. The reference PDw scan is shown for comparison, as well as the PSNR value.

Table 2. Results for inferring MR image contrasts (for 50 subjects). PSNR is computed for all different permutations of observed and missing contrasts. Results are shown as mean ± std.

Contrasts		PSNR		
Observed	Missing	T1w	T2w	PDw
T1w	T2w, PDw	-	28.9 ± 1.5	28.5 ± 1.1
T2w	T1w, PDw	28.2 ± 1.0	-	28.3 ± 1.5
PDw	T1w, T2w	28.0 ± 1.2	27.6 ± 1.6	-
T1w,T2w	PDw	-	-	28.8 ± 0.9
T2w,PDw	T1w	29.2 ± 1.4	-	-
T1w,PDw	T2w	-	28.1 ± 1.5	-

The example inferred PDw image in Fig. 3 looks realistic when compared to the known reference, although more noisy. The results in Table 2 are close to those previously reported in the literature [11] (for the same task but a different dataset).

3.2 MRI to CT Translation

Accurately translating MRIs to CTs is interesting for numerous reasons, *e.g.*, for removing the exposure to radiation that CT imaging involves, or for attenuation correction in MR-PET imaging. The proposed model should allow for this type of translation, by training it on subjects who have both MR and CT imaging. We therefore retrain the intensity distribution hyper-parameters of the model – retaining the template learnt from the IXI dataset – on eight patients from the RIRE dataset[5] [22]. Each patient in this dataset contains a number of imaging modalities. Here, only the patients with T1w and T2w MR scans (non-rectified), and CT images, are used. Note that the RIRE dataset is challenging to use due to the images having thick-slices, sometimes pathology, as well as requiring an initial co-registration (the dataset is part of a registration challenge and therefore purposefully misaligned). Each subject's scans are registered using the co-registration routine of the SPM12 software.

To test the models ability to translate MRIs to CTs, eight unseen RIRE patients are used[6]. The trained model is fit to each subject's T1w and T2w scans. The expected marginal posterior distribution over the missing CT image can then be computed. An example is shown in Fig. 4. The mean ± std PSNR between the inferred CT images and the known references is 25.5 ± 1.2. Considered the intensity hyper-parameters were trained on only eight subjects, the results are satisfactory, although not on pair with deep learning based techniques [13]. The

---

[5] https://www.insight-journal.org/rire/.
[6] The model is trained on RIRE patients `patient[102--109]`, and tested on `patient[001--007,101]`.

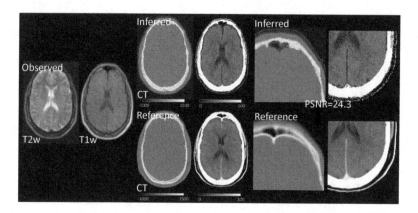

Fig. 4. Example of MRI to CT translation. An MR image with two channels (T1w and T2w) is observed. A CT scan is then inferred from the observed T1w and T2w scans. The reference CT scan is shown for comparison, as well as the PSNR value.

examples images in Fig. 4 suggests that the model does not capture a detailed enough distribution of bone. Additionally, the meninges does not appear in the inferred image, but is instead modelled as cerebrospinal fluid. Fitting not only the intensity hyper-parameters to the CT data, but also the template, could resolve these issues. More training data would also help.

4   Conclusion

This paper showed how a popular model for segmenting brain scans – a probabilistic forward model with a Gaussian mixture part – can be extended to infer missing data. For multi-channel segmentation, this extension circumvents the need to model only voxels that are observed in all channels. It furthermore enables predicting one MR contrast from another, or CTs from MRIs. The model gives reasonable results if trained on a small number of subjects, but we would expect further improvements with access to more training data. Interestingly, image translation is just a 'by-product' of learning the parameters of a joint probability distribution that models missing voxels. The same model can also be used to segment, bias correct and spatially normalise brain scans.

The model requires setting the number of Gaussian mixture components (K) at the start of the training. If this number is set too low, then the simulated images will look unrealistic. Here, this issue was resolved by using a fairly large number of components, which was found empirically capturing a detailed enough model distribution. Uninformative mixture components can then be drived to zero, due to the Bayesian setting of the Gaussian mixture model, by making point estimates of the values of the global tissue proportions (ω). This is known as automatic relevance determination [20].

Generative modelling approaches integrating multi-channel images, like the one presented here, should involve a component that relates signal across the various channels. The approach presented in this paper involves a probabilistic model of the relationship between signal intensities over channels. An alternative approach would be to use a multi-channel total variation (MTV) prior, which ensures that 'edges' appear in similar locations across channels. The MTV prior can be used to achieve super-resolution or denoising of medical images [23]. An avenue of future work could therefore be to incorporate both of these components into a super-resolution method, to improve resolution of thick-sliced, hospital-grade MR scans. By combining, for example, axial thick-sliced T2-weighted images and sagittal thick-sliced T1w images of the same subjects. In this example, the T2w image could provide some of the missing T1w signal in the left-right direction, whereas the T1w image could fill in some of the missing T2w signal in the inferior-posterior direction. Of course, this strategy would need to be formulated properly, but this work aimed to show a proof of the concept that one of those components, a probabilistic model between channels, does a good job at filling in missing data in MR images.

Acknowledgements. MB was funded by the EPSRC-funded UCL Centre for Doctoral Training in Medical Imaging (EP/L016478/1) and the Department of Health's NIHR-funded Biomedical Research Centre at University College London Hospitals. MB and JA was funded by the EU Human Brain Project's Grant Agreement No 785907 (SGA2). YB was funded by the MRC and Spinal Research Charity through the ERA-NET Neuron joint call (MR/R000050/1).

References

1. Burgos, N., et al.: Attenuation correction synthesis for hybrid PET-MR scanners. In: Mori, K., Sakuma, I., Sato, Y., Barillot, C., Navab, N. (eds.) MICCAI 2013. LNCS, vol. 8149, pp. 147–154. Springer, Heidelberg (2013). https://doi.org/10.1007/978-3-642-40811-3_19

2. Cao, T., Zach, C., Modla, S., Powell, D., Czymmek, K., Niethammer, M.: Registration for correlative microscopy using image analogies. In: Dawant, B.M., Christensen, G.E., Fitzpatrick, J.M., Rueckert, D. (eds.) WBIR 2012. LNCS, vol. 7359, pp. 296–306. Springer, Heidelberg (2012). https://doi.org/10.1007/978-3-642-31340-0_31

3. Roy, S., Carass, A., Shiee, N., Pham, D.L., Prince, J.L.: MR contrast synthesis for lesion segmentation. In: ISBI, pp. 932–935. IEEE (2010)

4. Kroon, D.-J., Slump, C.H.: MRI modalitiy transformation in demon registration. In: ISBI, pp. 963–966. IEEE (2009)

5. Guimond, A., Roche, A., Ayache, N., Meunier, J.: Three-dimensional multimodal brain warping using the demons algorithm and adaptive intensity corrections. IEEE Trans. Med. Imaging **20**(1), 58–69 (2001)

6. Wein, W., Brunke, S., Khamene, A., Callstrom, M.R., Navab, N.: Automatic CT-ultrasound registration for diagnostic imaging and image-guided intervention. Med. Image Anal. **12**(5), 577–585 (2008)

7. Hsu, S.-H., Cao, Y., Huang, K., Feng, M., Balter, J.M.: Investigation of a method for generating synthetic CT models from MRI scans of the head and neck for radiation therapy. Phys. Med. Biol. **58**(23), 8419 (2013)

8. Huynh, T., et al.: Estimating CT image from MRI data using structured random forest and auto-context model. IEEE Trans. Med. Imaging **35**(1), 174–183 (2015)
9. Iglesias, J.E., Konukoglu, E., Zikic, D., Glocker, B., Van Leemput, K., Fischl, B.: Is synthesizing MRI contrast useful for inter-modality analysis? In: Mori, K., Sakuma, I., Sato, Y., Barillot, C., Navab, N. (eds.) MICCAI 2013. LNCS, vol. 8149, pp. 631–638. Springer, Heidelberg (2013). https://doi.org/10.1007/978-3-642-40811-3_79
10. Roy, S., Carass, A., Prince, J.: A compressed sensing approach for MR tissue contrast synthesis. In: Székely, G., Hahn, H.K. (eds.) IPMI 2011. LNCS, vol. 6801, pp. 371–383. Springer, Heidelberg (2011). https://doi.org/10.1007/978-3-642-22092-0_31
11. Chartsias, A., Joyce, T., Giuffrida, M.V., Tsaftaris, S.A.: Multimodal MR synthesis via modality-invariant latent representation. IEEE Trans. Med. Imaging **37**(3), 803–814 (2017)
12. Nie, D., et al.: Medical image synthesis with context-aware generative adversarial networks. In: Descoteaux, M., Maier-Hein, L., Franz, A., Jannin, P., Collins, D.L., Duchesne, S. (eds.) MICCAI 2017. LNCS, vol. 10435, pp. 417–425. Springer, Cham (2017). https://doi.org/10.1007/978-3-319-66179-7_48
13. Wolterink, J.M., Dinkla, A.M., Savenije, M.H.F., Seevinck, P.R., van den Berg, C.A.T., Išgum, I.: Deep MR to CT synthesis using unpaired data. In: Tsaftaris, S.A., Gooya, A., Frangi, A.F., Prince, J.L. (eds.) SASHIMI 2017. LNCS, vol. 10557, pp. 14–23. Springer, Cham (2017). https://doi.org/10.1007/978-3-319-68127-6_2
14. Cohen, J.P., Luck, M., Honari, S.: Distribution matching losses can hallucinate features in medical image translation. In: Frangi, A.F., Schnabel, J.A., Davatzikos, C., Alberola-López, C., Fichtinger, G. (eds.) MICCAI 2018. LNCS, vol. 11070, pp. 529–536. Springer, Cham (2018). https://doi.org/10.1007/978-3-030-00928-1_60
15. Ghahramani, Z., Jordan, M.I.: Supervised learning from incomplete data via an EM approach. In: NeurIPS, pp. 120–127 (1994)
16. Ashburner, J., Friston, K.J.: Unified segmentation. Neuroimage **26**(3), 839–851 (2005)
17. Blaiotta, C., Freund, P., Cardoso, M.J., Ashburner, J.: Generative diffeomorphic modelling of large MRI data sets for probabilistic template construction. Neuroimage **166**, 117–134 (2018)
18. Carlin, B.P., Louis, T.A.: Empirical bayes: past, present and future. J. Am. Stat. Assoc. **95**(452), 1286–1289 (2000)
19. Blaiotta, C., Cardoso, M.J., Ashburner, J.: Variational inference for medical image segmentation. Comput. Vis. Image Underst. **151**, 14–28 (2016)
20. Bishop, C.M.: Pattern Recognition and Machine Learning. Springer, Heidelberg (2006)
21. Brudfors, M., Balbastre, Y., Ashburner, J.: Nonlinear Markov random fields learned via backpropagation. In: Chung, A.C.S., Gee, J.C., Yushkevich, P.A., Bao, S. (eds.) IPMI 2019. LNCS, vol. 11492, pp. 805–817. Springer, Cham (2019). https://doi.org/10.1007/978-3-030-20351-1_63
22. West, J.B., Woods, R.P.: Comparison and evaluation of retrospective intermodality image registration techniques. In: Medical Imaging 1996: Image Processing, vol. 2710, pp. 332–348. SPIE (1996)
23. Brudfors, M., Balbastre, Y., Nachev, P., Ashburner, J.: MRI super-resolution using multi-channel total variation. In: Nixon, M., Mahmoodi, S., Zwiggelaar, R. (eds.) MIUA 2018. CCIS, vol. 894, pp. 217–228. Springer, Cham (2018). https://doi.org/10.1007/978-3-319-95921-4_21

Improved MR to CT Synthesis
for PET/MR Attenuation Correction
Using Imitation Learning

Kerstin Kläser[1,2]([✉]), Thomas Varsavsky[1,2], Pawel Markiewicz[1,2],
Tom Vercauteren[2], David Atkinson[4], Kris Thielemans[3], Brian Hutton[3],
M. Jorge Cardoso[2], and Sébastien Ourselin[2]

[1] Department of Medical Physics and Biomedical Engineering,
University College London, London, UK
`kerstin.klaser.16@ucl.ac.uk`
[2] School of Biomedical Engineering and Imaging Sciences,
King's College London, London, UK
[3] Institute of Nuclear Medicine, University College London, London, UK
[4] Centre for Medical Imaging, University College London, London, UK

Abstract. The ability to synthesise Computed Tomography images -
commonly known as pseudo CT, or pCT - from MRI input data is commonly assessed using an intensity-wise similarity, such as an L_2-norm
between the ground truth CT and the pCT. However, given that the
ultimate purpose is often to use the pCT as an attenuation map (μ-
map) in Positron Emission Tomography Magnetic Resonance Imaging
(PET/MRI), minimising the error between pCT and CT is not necessarily optimal. The main objective should be to predict a pCT that,
when used as μ-map, reconstructs a pseudo PET (pPET) which is as
close as possible to the gold standard PET. To this end, we propose a
novel multi-hypothesis deep learning framework that generates pCTs by
minimising a combination of the pixel-wise error between pCT and CT
and a proposed metric-loss that itself is represented by a convolutional
neural network (CNN) and aims to minimise subsequent PET residuals. The model is trained on a database of 400 paired MR/CT/PET
image slices. Quantitative results show that the network generates pCTs
that seem less accurate when evaluating the Mean Absolute Error on
the pCT (69.68HU) compared to a baseline CNN (66.25HU), but lead to
significant improvement in the PET reconstruction - 115$a.u.$ compared
to baseline 140$a.u.$

1 Introduction

The combination of Positron Emission Tomography (PET) and Magnetic Resonance Imaging (MRI) marked a significant event in the field of Nuclear Medicine,
facilitating simultaneous structural and functional characterisation of soft tissue
[1]. In order to accurately reconstruct quantitative PET images, it is indispensable to correct for attenuation of the whole imaging object (part of the human

© Springer Nature Switzerland AG 2019
N. Burgos et al. (Eds.): SASHIMI 2019, LNCS 11827, pp. 13–21, 2019.
https://doi.org/10.1007/978-3-030-32778-1_2

body) including the hardware (patient bed and additional coils). However, this is particularly challenging in PET/MRI as there is no direct correlation between MR image intensities and attenuation coefficients in contrast to the case when a CT image is available. In hybrid imaging systems that combine PET with Computed Tomography (CT), the tissue density information is derived from the CT image as Hounsfield units (HU), which can bi-linear approximate the attenuation coefficients (μ). While CT remains the clinically accepted gold-standard for PET/MR attenuation correction, it is desirable to generate accurate μ-maps without the need for an additional CT acquisition. Hence, the concept of synthesising pseudo CT (pCT) images from MRs raised significant attention in the research area of PET/MR reconstruction.

Recently, a multi-centre study has shown that compared to physics and segmentation based approaches, methods based on multi-atlas approaches were best suited to generate appropriate pCTs. These methods estimate μ-maps on a continuous scale by deforming an anatomical model that contains paired MR and CT data to match the subject's anatomy by using non-rigid registration algorithms [2].

In recent years, there has been a shift of emphasis in the field of PET/MR attenuation correction towards deep learning approaches that have demonstrated significant improvements in the MR to CT image translation task, surpassing state-of-the-art multi-atlas-based approaches [3]. Such methods often utilise convolutional neural networks (CNN) that are able to capture the contextual information between two image domains (as between MR and CT) in order to translate one possible representation of an image into another. Supervised learning settings assume that the training dataset comprises examples of an input image (e.g. MR here) along with their corresponding target image (i.e. CT here). A popular method to optimise image translation networks is to minimise the residuals between the predicted pCT and the corresponding ground-truth CT, equivalent to minimising the $\mathcal{L}_2$-loss. $\mathcal{L}_2$-losses make sense when the optimal pCT for PET reconstruction is the one that is the closest, intensity-wise, to the target ground truth CT. However, this $\mathcal{L}_2$-loss fails to recognise that the primary objective of CT synthesis is to create a synthetic CT that, when used to reconstruct the PET image, makes it as close as possible to the gold standard PET reconstructed with the true CT. Also, the risk-minimising nature of the $\mathcal{L}_2$-loss disregards the fact that small local differences between the pCT and the true CT can have a large impact on the reconstructed PET. This downstream impact in PET reconstruction is illustrated in Fig. 1.

With the emergence of the cycleGAN in 2017 [4], many efforts have been made to synthesise CT images in an unsupervised manner disregarding the need of the $\mathcal{L}_2$-loss. Wolterink et al. [5] used a CNN that minimises an adversarial loss to learn the mapping from MR to CT. This adversarial loss forces the pseudo CT to be indistinguishable from a real CT. A second CNN ensures that the pseudo CT corresponds to the actual input MR image. However, using a cycleGAN only to synthesise pseudo CTs does not necessarily guarantee structural consistency between pseudo CT and original CT. Therefore Yang et al. [6] proposed

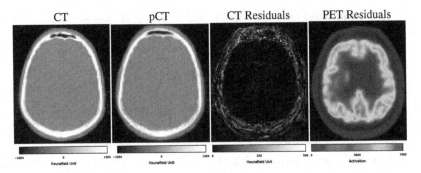

Fig. 1. (a) The ground truth CT, (b) the predicted pseudo CT, (c) the absolute residual between true and pseudo CT, and (d) the absolute residual between PETs reconstructed using the CT and synthetic CT as attenuation maps. Note that small and very localised difference in the CT (c) result in large PET residuals (d). We argue that algorithms should be optimising for PET residuals (d) and not for CT residuals (c).

a structure-constraint cycleGAN that minimises an additional structural consistency loss. In 2019, Jin et al. [7] presented a method that combines paired and unpaired data in order to overcome the missing structural consistency of the cycleGAN and to mitigate the errors introduced by the registration of paired data.

To the best of our knowledge, all these methods focus on minimising the error of the synthesised pCT. However, synthesising a CT image only acts as an interim step when aiming for PET attenuation correction creating an additional stage for potentially introduced errors. This work aims to directly minimise the PET residuals and achieves this by introducing a novel MR to CT synthesis framework that is composed of two separate CNNs. The first network generates multiple plausible CT representations using Multi-Hypothesis Learning instead of just a single pCT [8]. An oracle determines the most correct predictor and only updates the weights with regards to the winning mode, enabling the first network to specialise in generating pCTs with specific features (e.g. skull thickness, bone density). A second network then predicts the residuals between ground-truth PETs and PETs reconstructed using each plausible pCT using imitation learning. In this setting, the second network can be seen as a metric that estimates the pPET residuals, and thus, by minimising this metric, the network learns to generate pCTs that will subsequently result in pPETs with lower residual errors.

2   Methods

2.1   Multi-hypothesis Learning

Given a set of input MR images $x \in \mathcal{X}$ and a set of output CT images $y \in \mathcal{Y}$, the proposed image synthesis approach aims to find a mapping function f_ϕ between the two image domains $\mathcal{X}$ and $\mathcal{Y}$, i.e. $f_\phi : \mathcal{X} \to \mathcal{Y}$ with unique parameters

$\phi \in \mathbb{R}^n$. In a supervised learning setting with a set of N paired training tuples (x_i, y_i), $i = 1, ..., N$, we try to find the predictor f_ϕ that minimises the error

$$\frac{1}{N} \sum_{i=1}^{N} \mathcal{L}(f_\phi(x_i), y_i).$$

where $\mathcal{L}$ can be any desired loss, such as the classical $\mathcal{L}_2$-loss. In the proposed multi-hypothesis scenario, the network provides multiple predictions pCT, where $f_\phi^j(x) \in (f_\phi^1(x), ..., f_\phi^M(x))$ with $M \in \mathbb{N}$.

As in the original work [8], only the loss of the best predictor $f_\phi^j(x)$ will be considered in the training following a Winner-Takes-All (WTA) strategy, i.e.

$$\mathcal{L}(f_\phi(x_i), y_i) = min_{j \in [1,M]} \mathcal{L}(f_\phi^j(x_i), y_i).$$

This way the network learns M modes to predict pCTs each specialising on specific features.

2.2   Imitation Learning

Following the hypothesis that the $\mathcal{L}_2$-loss is not an optimal loss metric when generating pCTs for the purpose of PET/MR attenuation correction because of its risk minimising nature, we propose to train a second network that, by taking ground truth CTs (y_i) and pCTs $(f_\phi^j(x_i) \in \tilde{\mathcal{Y}})$ as inputs, aims to approximate the function $g_\psi : \mathcal{Y}, \tilde{\mathcal{Y}} \rightarrow \mathcal{Z}$ with $\psi \in \mathbb{R}^n$. Here, $\mathcal{Z}$ is a set of error maps between the ground truth PET and the pPET that was reconstructed using each of the M pCT realisations as μ-maps. In other words, this second network tries to predict what the PET residuals would be from an input CT-pCT pair, thus imitating, or approximating, the PET reconstruction process. We train this imitation network by minimising the $\mathcal{L}_2$-loss between the true PET uptake error z and the predicted error $\tilde{z}$, i.e. $\mathcal{L}_2 = ||z - \tilde{z}||_2$.

Lastly, we use this second network as a new loss function for the first network, as it provides an approximate and differentiable estimate of the PET residual loss. The loss minimised by the first network is then defined as $\mathcal{L}(x_i, y_i, z_i) = min_{m \in [1,M]}[g_\psi(f_\phi(x_i), y_i), z_i]$.

2.3   Proposed Network Architecture

The proposed network architecture (Fig. 2) is trained in three phases: First, a HighResNet [9] with multiple hypothesis outputs is trained with $\mathcal{L}_2$-WTA loss to generate different pCT (yellow box). In the second stage, while freezing the weights of the first network a second instance (purple box) of HighResNet is trained to learn the error prediction between true and predicted PET and learn the mapping between pCT residual and subsequent pPET reconstruction error. Once learnt, the first network is retrained using both the CT $\mathcal{L}_2$-loss and the metric loss in equal proportions.

2.4   Implementation Details

The training was performed on whole images using 70% of the dataset (10% was reserved for validation and 20% for testing). All training phases were performed on a Titan V GPU with Adam optimiser. A model was trained with a learning rate of 0.001 for 20k iterations decreasing the learning rate by a factor of 10 and resuming training until convergence. The architecture was implemented using NiftyNet, an open-source TensorFlow-based CNN platform developed for research in the domain of medical image analysis [10].

3   Experimental Datasets and Materials

The experimental dataset consisted of pairs of T1- and T2-weighted MR and CT brain images of 20 patients. For each subject, an intra-subject registration was performed, where MRs and CTs were aligned using first a rigid registration algorithm followed by a very low degree of freedom non-rigid deformation [3]. A second non-linear registration was performed, using a cubic B-spline with normalised mutual information, only on the neck region to correct for soft tissue shift [11]. Each volume had $301 \times 301 \times 153$ voxels with a voxel size of approximately $1 \, mm^3$. For the purpose of this work, the original data was then resampled to the original Siemens Biograph mMR PET resolution of $344 \times 344 \times 127$ voxels with a voxel size of approximately $2 \, mm^3$ before we extracted the 20 central slices per

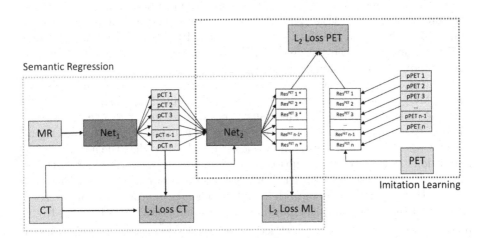

Fig. 2. Yellow box: semantic regression. Net_1 takes MR images as inputs and predicts multiple pCT realisations by minimising a combination of the $\mathcal{L}_2$-loss between ground truth CT and pCT ($\mathcal{L}_2$-loss CT) and a learned metric loss ($\mathcal{L}_2$-loss ML). In the first stage only $\mathcal{L}_2$-loss CT is considered and $\mathcal{L}_2$-loss ML is weighted to zero. Purple box: imitation network. Net_2 takes pCTs and corresponding CTs as input and predicts the error between ground truth PET and pPET reconstructed with pCT as μ-map by minimising $\mathcal{L}_2$-loss PET. Semantic regression and imitation network are trained separately in three stages. (Color figure online)

volume resulting in a registered 2D MR/CT/PET dataset of 400 images. MR and CT images were downsampled because all image analysis was performed in the original PET space since the ultimate aim of the method is to minimise PET residuals. For evaluation purposes, a head region mask was extracted from the CT image to exclude the background from the performance metric analysis. In order to train the imitation network, three PETs were reconstructed using each of the multi-hypothesis pCTs over 20 slices (here denoted as pPET), resulting in a total of 60 pCT/pPET pairs. PET reconstruction was performed using NiftyPET [12]. Since the raw PET data was not accessible, the following simulation was performed: a PET forward projection was applied on the μ-map transformed versions of the pCTs in order to obtain attenuation factor sinograms. Similar forward projection was applied to the original PET images to obtain simulated emission sinograms which are then attenuated through element-wise multiplication using the attenuation factor sinograms. Those simulated sinograms were then reconstructed using both the original CT-based attenuation map to obtain a reference image, as well as the attenuation maps derived from the different pCT images.

4   Experiments and Results

Qualitative results are presented in Fig. 3. The first column shows the ground truth CT image (top), the pCTs generated with the HighResNet that we used as baseline (middle) and a pCT generated with the proposed imitation learning (bottom). Next to the CTs (2nd column) the error between pCT and ground truth CT is shown. In the third column the true PET (top), imitation learning pPET (middle) and the baseline pPET (bottom) are shown followed by the corresponding pPET residuals in the last column.

As a second experiment, we performed an evaluation on the use of Monte-Carlo (MC) dropout versus multi-hypothesis as a sampling scheme to generate multiple realisations of pCTs. The results are depicted in Fig. 4. The variance in the pPET intensities, which was reconstructed with a μ-map from the pCTs generated with MC dropout, was found to be artificially low, while the multiple pCT realisations of the proposed multi-hypothesis model provided a wider distribution of pPET intensities. In order to investigate the accuracy of the predictions, we investigated the Z-score of both sampling schemes in order to show the relationship of the mean data distribution to the ground truth PET. Figure 4-Right presents the per pixel Z-score defined as $\frac{\text{PET}-\mu(\text{pPET}^M)}{\sigma(\text{pPET}^M)}$, with $\mu(\text{pPET}^M)$ and $\sigma(\text{pPET}^M)$ being the per-pixel average and per pixel variance over M pPET samples respectively. Results show that the Z-score for multi-hypothesis is significantly lower in the brain region than the one from MC dropout, meaning that the multi-hypothesis-based PET uncertainty does encompass the true PET value more often than the competing MC dropout method.

In a third experiment, and for quantification purposes, we calculated the Mean Absolute Error (MAE) of the pseudo CTs only in the head region

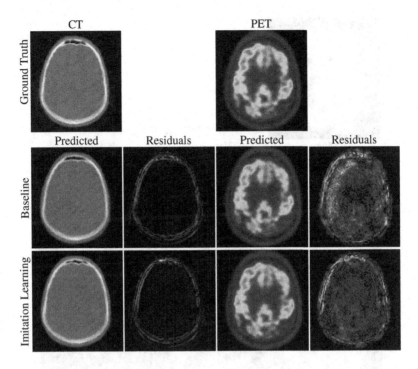

Fig. 3. Qualitative results. From top to bottom: Ground-truth, baseline (HighResNet), and imitation learning. From left to right: CT, pCT-CT residuals, PET, pPET-PET residuals. As expected, we note that MAE in the pCT generated with the proposed imitation learning is higher than the baseline, but the resulting pPET error is significantly *lower* for the proposed method.

and of the pseudo PET only in the brain region by masking out the background of the images. We validated the advantages of the proposed imitation learning model on the remaining 20% of the dataset hold out for testing (see Table 1). Although, as expected, the proposed method leads to a higher MAE on the CT (69.68 ± 32.22HU) compared to the simple feed forward model (66.25 ± 30.54HU), the MAE in the resulting pPET is significantly lower (paired t-test, $p < 10^{-4}$) for the proposed method (115.41 ± 78.72) when compared to the baseline model (140.76 ± 91.87). The proposed method also outperforms the multi-hypothesis only approach in both metrics.

5   Discussion and Conclusion

In this work, we proposed a novel network architecture for pCT synthesis for PET/MR attenuation correction. We were able to show that the $\mathcal{L}_2$-loss, often used as a minimisation metric in the field of CT synthesis, is not optimal when ultimately aiming for a low error in the corresponding pPET when used as attenuation map. Quantitative analysis on an independent dataset confirmed the

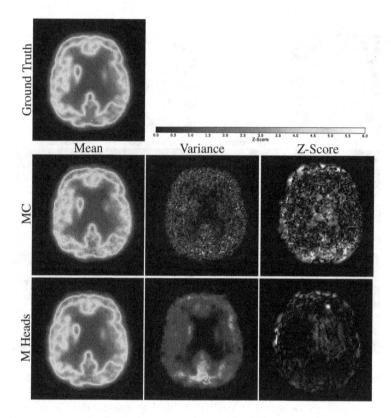

Fig. 4. PET intensities (first column), variance (middle column) and Z-score (right column) of ground truth PET (top row) compared to pPET intensities reconstructed with pCTs from Monte Carlo (MC) dropout sampling (middle row) and pCTs from multi-hypothesis sampling (bottom row). Sampling from multi-hypothesis captures true PET intensities better than sampling from MC dropout.

Table 1. Mean Absolute Error (MAE) pCTs generated with HighResNet, Multi-hypothesis pCTs and Imitation Learning pCTs and corresponding MAE in pPET.

Method	MAE CT (in HU)	MAE PET (in a.u.)
HighResNet	66.25 ± 30.54	140.76 ± 91.87
Multi-hypothesis	72.23 ± 27.69	215.57 ± 102.99
Imitation learning	69.68 ± 32.22	115.41 ± 78.72

proposed hypothesis that pCTs with a low MAE do not necessarily result in a low pPET error. This work also demonstrates that minimising a more suitable metric that indeed optimises for PET residuals (from CTs and pCTs) can improve the process of CT synthesis for PET/MR attenuation correction.

Acknowledgment. This work was supported by an IMPACT studentship funded jointly by Siemens and the EPSRC UCL CDT in Medical Imaging (EP/L016478/1). We gratefully acknowledge the support of NVIDIA Corporation with the donation of one Titan V. This project has received funding from Wellcome Flagship Programme (WT213038/Z/18/Z), the Wellcome EPSRC CME (WT203148/Z/16/Z), the NIHR GSTT Biomedical Research Centre, and the NIHR UCLH Biomedical Research Centre.

References

1. Pichler, B.J., et al.: Positron emission tomography/magnetic resonance imaging: the next generation of multimodality imaging? In: Seminars in Nuclear Medicine, vol. 38, pp. 199–208. Elsevier (2008)
2. Ladefoged, C.N., et al.: A multi-centre evaluation of eleven clinically feasible brain PET/MRI attenuation correction techniques using a large cohort of patients. Neuroimage **147**, 346–359 (2017)
3. Burgos, N., et al.: Attenuation correction synthesis for hybrid PET-MR scanners: application to brain studies. IEEE TMI **33**(12), 2332–2341 (2014)
4. Zhu, J.Y., et al.: Unpaired image-to-image translation using cycle-consistent adversarial networks. arXiv preprint arXiv:1703.10593 (2017)
5. Wolterink, J.M., Dinkla, A.M., Savenije, M.H.F., Seevinck, P.R., van den Berg, C.A.T., Išgum, I.: Deep MR to CT synthesis using unpaired data. In: Tsaftaris, S.A., Gooya, A., Frangi, A.F., Prince, J.L. (eds.) SASHIMI 2017. LNCS, vol. 10557, pp. 14–23. Springer, Cham (2017). https://doi.org/10.1007/978-3-319-68127-6_2
6. Yang, H., et al.: Unpaired brain MR-to-CT synthesis using a structure-constrained CycleGAN. In: Stoyanov, D., et al. (eds.) DLMIA/ML-CDS -2018. LNCS, vol. 11045, pp. 174–182. Springer, Cham (2018). https://doi.org/10.1007/978-3-030-00889-5_20
7. Jin, C.B., et al.: Deep CT to MR synthesis using paired and unpaired data. Sensors **19**(10), 2361 (2019)
8. Rupprecht, C., et al.: Learning in an uncertain world: representing ambiguity through multiple hypotheses. In: Proceedings of the IEEE ICCV, pp. 3591–3600 (2017)
9. Li, W., Wang, G., Fidon, L., Ourselin, S., Cardoso, M.J., Vercauteren, T.: On the compactness, efficiency, and representation of 3D convolutional networks: brain parcellation as a pretext task. In: Niethammer, M., et al. (eds.) IPMI 2017. LNCS, vol. 10265, pp. 348–360. Springer, Cham (2017). https://doi.org/10.1007/978-3-319-59050-9_28
10. Gibson, E., et al.: NiftyNet: a deep-learning platform for medical imaging. CoRR abs/1709.03485 (2017)
11. Modat, M., et al.: Fast free-form deformation using graphics processing units. Comput. Methods Programs Biomed. **98**(3), 278–284 (2010)
12. Markiewicz, P.J., et al.: NiftyPET: a high-throughput software platform for high quantitative accuracy and precision PET imaging and analysis. Neuroinformatics **16**(1), 95–115 (2018)

Unpaired Multi-contrast MR Image Synthesis Using Generative Adversarial Networks

Muhammad Sohail[1], Muhammad Naveed Riaz[2], Jing Wu[1(✉)], Chengnian Long[1], and Shaoyuan Li[1]

[1] Department of Automation and Key Laboratory of System Control and Information Processing, Ministry of Education of China, Shanghai Jiaotong University, Shanghai 200240, China
{sohail_sjtu,jingwu}@sjtu.edu.cn
[2] Department of Computer Science, Shanghai Jiao Tong University, Shanghai 200240, China

Abstract. Magnetic Resonance Imaging (MRI) has been established as an important diagnostic tool for research and clinical purposes. Multi-contrast scans can enhance the accuracy for many deep learning algorithms. However, these scans may not be available in some situations. Thus, it is valuable to synthetically generate non-existent contrasts from the available one. Existing methods based on Generative Adversarial Networks (GANs) lack the freedom to map one image to multiple contrasts using only a single generator and discriminator, hence, requiring training of multiple models for multi-contrast MR synthesis. We present a novel method for multi-contrast MR image synthesis with unpaired data using GANs. Our method leverages the strength of Star-GAN to translate a given image to n contrasts using a single generator and discriminator. We also introduce a new generation loss function, which enforces the generator to produce high-quality images which are perceptually closer to the real ones and exhibit high structural similarity as well. We experiment on IXI dataset to learn all possible mappings among T_1-weighted, T_2-weighted, Proton Density (PD) weighted and Magnetic Resonance Angiography (MRA) images. Qualitative and quantitative comparison against baseline method shows the superiority of our approach.

Keywords: Generative Adversarial Networks · Multi-contrast synthesis · MR Imaging

1 Introduction

Within last three and a half decade Magnetic Resonance Imaging (MRI) has evolved from a potential idea to primary diagnostic tool for many clinical and

This work was supported by National Natural Science Foundation (NNSF) of China under Grant 61873166, 61673275 and 61473184.

N. Burgos et al. (Eds.): SASHIMI 2019, LNCS 11827, pp. 22–31, 2019.
https://doi.org/10.1007/978-3-030-32778-1_3

research problems [1]. The reason for such an enormous growth is its non-invasive nature, the ability to generate distinct contrasts of same anatomical structure and non-exposure to ionization radiation [2]. Different deep learning methods utilize these multi-contrast MR images (T_1-weighted, T_2-weighted etc.,) for brain tumor segmentation [3] and white/gray matter segmentation [4]. However, these deep neural networks rely heavily on huge datasets for training. The availability of such datasets in the domain of medical imaging is quite challenging and it becomes even more difficult when the required data is multi-contrast. Therefore, to enhance the performance of deep learning methods, synthetic generation of images for data augmentation is of great importance [5].

Since the introduction of generative adversarial networks (GANs), there has been remarkable development in the direction of image synthesis [6]. GANs have been widely adopted in medical imaging, [5] uses Wasserstein-GANs to generate T_1-weighted, T_2-weighted and FLAIR images of brain, [3] used Progressively Growing GANs for generation of retinal fundus and brain images. Some cross-modality image synthesis methods based on Cycle-GAN [7], cGAN [8] and Pix2Pix [9] have also been presented for generating missing modality data. However, all of these methods are limited to generate synthetic data for one or two contrasts only. For generation of multi-contrast data, existing methods require training of separate models for each corresponding contrast which is extensively time consuming, and computationally very expensive. This also limits the potential of generator network to learn common features from all available data samples which is crucial when training dataset is small.

To alleviate the above issue, we propose a new method, which leverages the power of Star-GAN [6] and U-NET [10] for synthetic generation of multi-contrast MR images (T_1-weighted, T_2-weighted, PD-weighted and MRA) using only one generator and discriminator network. Our method eliminates the requirement of training separate models for each mapping, thus, reducing the training time significantly. In addition, our approach allows us to utilize images from all contrasts for training in an unsupervised manner, which helps the generator to learn common geometric properties among all contrasts. The unsupervised training eliminates the requirement of paired data, hence broadening the scope of our method.

A new generation loss is proposed which preserves the small anatomical structural details of given input image using structural similarity (SSIM) [11]. It also employs recently proposed Learned Perceptual Image Patch Similarity (LPIPS) metric [12], that forces the generator to learn reverse mapping for reconstructing real image from fake image while prioritizing perceptual similarity between reconstructed and real images. For stable training of our model we add regularization term to the adversarial loss [13]. The model is trained to generate images for all four contrasts using only one image as input from any contrast. We provide qualitative and quantitative results for synthetic generation of multi-contrast MR images, which shows the superiority of our approach over existing methods.

2 Method

The proposed method efficiently and effectively learns the mappings among four contrasts of MRI [T_1-weighted, T_2-weighted, Proton Density (PD)-weighted, Magnetic Resonance Angiography (MRA)] to generate a fake image of target contrast given a real image and original contrast. For example, given an input image of T_1-weighted contrast our model can generate fake T_2-weighted, PD-weighted and MRA images using only one generator. Working of the model is illustrated by Fig. 1 and details of loss functions are described next.

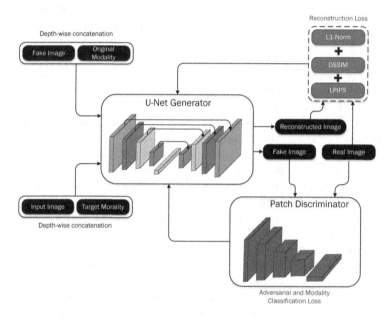

Fig. 1. U-NET generator performs two synthesis: (i) generating a fake image given depth-wise concatenated real image and target contrast; (ii) reconstructing real image given fake image concatenated depth-wise with original contrast. Fake image is used to measure two losses: (i) Adversarial loss and (ii) contrast classification loss using Patch-GAN discriminator. Reconstructed and real image are used to measure reconstruction loss to observe how close reconstructed image is to the real image in terms of structural (SSIM), perceptual (LPIPS) and global (L_1) similarity

2.1 Loss Functions

Adversarial Loss: Instead of using adversarial loss proposed by [14], which is reported to suffer from various training problems including mode collapse, vanishing gradients and senstitivity to hyper-parameters, we use regularized Wassersteing GAN with gradient penalty (WGAN-GP). This not only provides stable learning for deep generator and discriminator networks but also increase the quality of generated images. It is defined as

$$\mathcal{L}_{adv} = \mathcal{L}_{WGAN_{gp}} + \lambda_{ct} CT|_{x',x''} \tag{1}$$

Here, the first term gives us the WGAN-GP loss and the second term regularize this loss using a consistency term. WGAN-GP loss is given as

$$\mathcal{L}_{WGAN_{gp}} = \mathbb{E}\big[D_{src}(x)\big] - \mathbb{E}_{x,c}\big[D_{src}(G(x,c))\big]$$
$$-\lambda_{gp}\mathbb{E}_{\hat{x}}\big[(\|\nabla_{\hat{x}} D_{src}(\hat{x})\|_2 - 1)^2\big] \tag{2}$$

In above equation, generator G takes an input image x and a target label c to generate a fake image of the target contrast. While the discriminator D is responsible for finding out if the given image is real (from training set) or fake (generated by G). The consistency term of Eq. 1 is given as

$$CT|_{x',x''} = \mathbb{E}_{x\sim\mathbb{P}}\big[max(0, d(D(x'), D(x'')))$$
$$+0.1 \cdot d(D_-(x'), D_-(x'')) - M')\big] \tag{3}$$

here, x' and x'' corresponds to virtual data points close to x and D_- is the output of the discriminator from second to the last layer.

For our experiments, we use $\lambda_{gp} = 10$, $\lambda_{ct} = 1$ and $M' = 0$.

Contrast Classification Loss: It forces the generator to produce image of correct contrast and allows discriminator to perform contrast classification for real and fake images [6]. It is defined as

$$\mathcal{L}_{cls}^r = \mathbb{E}_{x,c'}\big[-\log D_{cls}(c'|x)\big] \tag{4}$$

for fake images

$$\mathcal{L}_{cls}^f = \mathbb{E}_{x,c'}\big[-\log D_{cls}(c'|G(x,c)\big] \tag{5}$$

Here, x and c' represents real image and original label. while $G(x,c)$ and c corresponds to fake image and target contrast.

Generation Loss: If the model generates a fake image T_1' belonging to T_1 contrast using a real T_2-weighted image then by using reverse mapping it should reconstruct the real T_2-weighted image. For this [7] uses cycle consistency loss:

$$\mathcal{L}_{cyc} = \mathbb{E}_{x,c,c'}\big[\|x - G(G(x,c), c')\|\big] \tag{6}$$

However, this L_1 loss focuses on an entire image ignoring patch level dissimilarity among images, thus providing less information for generator to work with. Therefore, to impose small patch wise dissimilarity measure between real and reconstructed image, we increment generation loss with two additional terms. (i) Inspired by the strength of structural similarity (SSIM) [11] for measuring structural similarity between two images in a patch-wise manner, we employ structural dissimilarity loss (DSSIM); an extension of (SSIM) as

$$\mathcal{L}_{DSSIM} = \mathbb{E}_{x,c,c'}\left[\frac{1 - SSIM(x - G(G(x,c), c'))}{2}\right] \tag{7}$$

(ii) Secondly, to enforce the generator to produce images perpetually more closer to the target contrast, we utilize recently proposed Learned Perceptual Image Patch Similarity metric [12]:

$$\mathcal{L}_{LPIPS} = \mathbb{E}_{x,c,c'} \left[x - G(G(x,c),c') \right] \tag{8}$$

Both additional terms calculate differences between real and reconstructed image in a patch wise manner. This allows our generator to focus on small anatomical regions and preserve structure while changing only contrast related properties for image synthesis. Our final reconstruction loss takes the good from all three terms:

$$\mathcal{L}_{rec} = \lambda_{cyc} \mathcal{L}_{cyc} + \lambda_{DSSIM} \mathcal{L}_{DSSIM} + \lambda_{lpips} \mathcal{L}_{lpips} \tag{9}$$

We use $\lambda_{cyc} = \lambda_{DSSIM} = \lambda_{lpips} = 10$ for training.

Full Objective: Finally, the full objective for our discriminator network is to minimize the loss $\mathcal{L}_D$, which is defined as

$$\mathcal{L}_D = -\mathcal{L}_{adv} + \mathcal{L}_{cls}^r \tag{10}$$

while the generator tries to minimize $\mathcal{L}_G$ given as

$$\mathcal{L}_G = \mathcal{L}_{adv} + \mathcal{L}_{cls}^f + \mathcal{L}_{rec} \tag{11}$$

2.2   Network Architecture

For the exceptional performance of U-Net [10] for medical images, we use U-Net based generator for our model adapted from [7]. The generator contains 7 down-sampling layers with strided convolutions of stride 2 followed by the 7 up-sampling layers with fractional strides. Each convolutional layer is followed by instance normalization and ReLU activation except for the final layer which uses tanh after convolution layer. Similar to [6,7,15] we are using PatchGANs-based discriminator which can classify local patches for real or fake, providing efficiency over full image classifier. No normalization is applied to discriminator.

3   Experiments and Results

3.1   Dataset

We use IXI dataset[1] for all of our experiments, which provides scans of almost 600 subjects for all four contrasts. Images for IXI dataset are acquired using three different scanners, however information for only two (Philips Medical Systems Gyroscan Intera 1.5T $\rightarrow$ $S1$, Philips Medical Systems Intera 3T $\rightarrow$ $S2$)is available which is provided in Table 1. Since, the provided images were not registered we used AntsPy[2] package for registering all images to a common template using affine transformation. This provides us with 568 images of same size and position from which 68 were randomly selected for testing while remaining 500 were used for training. Since the MRA images of IXI dataset provide better resolution in axial plane, therefore, axial slices of all images were taken.

---

[1] https://brain-development.org/ixi-dataset/.
[2] https://github.com/ANTsX/ANTsPy.

Table 1. Images acquisition parameters

Dimensions	T_1-weighted	T_2-weighted	PD-weighted	MRA
Flip Anlge$_{S1}$	8	90	90	25
Flip Anlge$_{S2}$	8	90	90	16
TE$_{S1}$	4.6 ms	100 ms	8 ms	6.9 ms
TE$_{S2}$	4.6 ms	100 ms	8 ms	5.75 ms
TR$_{S1}$	9.813 ms	8178.34 ms	8178.34 ms	20 ms
TR$_{S2}$	9.60 ms	5725.79 ms	5725.79.34 ms	20 ms
Volume Size	$256 \times 256 \times 150$	$256 \times 256 \times 130$	$256 \times 256 \times 130$	$512 \times 512 \times 100$
Voxel Dimensions	$0.94 \times 0.94 \times 1.2$	$0.94 \times 0.94 \times 1.2$	$0.94 \times 0.94 \times 1.2$	$0.47 \times 0.47 \times 0.8$

3.2 Implementation Details

For all of our experiments we used PyTorch, and the image slices were center croped and resized to 256×256 due to computational limitations. Input image and target contrast are selected randomly in an unpaired manner for training. For fair comparison both models default Star-GAN and proposed use same values of hyperparameters. Both models are trained for 200,000 iterations with a batch size of 10, for optimization Adam optimizer with momentum of 0.9 is used.

3.3 Quantitative Results

To evaluate the performance of our model against Star-GAN, we utilize the commonly used metrics of peak signal-noise ratio (PSNR), SSIM [11] and LPIPS [12]. The averaged results of 4129 slices for each meaningful mapping are shown in Table 2. Here, high PSNR, SSIM and lower LPIPS means better quality of the generated images. Our method has clearly outperformed Star-GAN for all mappings.

3.4 Qualitative Results

Figures 2, 3 and 4 shows the qualitative comparison of our method against Star-GAN for multi-contrast synthesis. It can be seen that images generated by Star-GAN lack structural and perceptual similarity for small anatomical regions, which are captured by our method. Synthesis of MRA from T_2-weighted image Fig. 2 shows Star-GAN failed to capture the overall color of the image, while our method generated image identical to the real one. Similarly Figs. 3 and 4 show the superiority of our method.

Table 2. Synthesis: Real Image → Fake Image (generated by network).

Mappings	Star-GAN			Proposed Method		
	PSNR	SSIM	LPIPS	PSNR	SSIM	LPIPS
$T_2 \rightarrow$ MRA	19.51	0.4502	0.1628	**27.17**	**0.7545**	**0.0688**
$T_2 \rightarrow$ PD	21.81	0.7882	0.0614	**25.30**	**0.9118**	**0.0287**
$T_2 \rightarrow T_1$	18.46	0.6135	0.0902	**20.05**	**0.6864**	**0.0650**
MRA $\rightarrow$ PD	20.66	0.6197	0.1152	**22.43**	**0.7345**	**0.0694**
MRA $\rightarrow T_1$	20.34	0.7169	0.1032	**21.78**	**0.8016**	**0.0698**
MRA $\rightarrow T_2$	20.81	0.6373	0.1211	**20.90**	**0.7106**	**0.0680**
PD $\rightarrow$ MRA	16.02	0.4182	0.1817	**25.18**	**0.7348**	**0.0648**
PD $\rightarrow T_1$	18.81	0.6352	0.0842	**21.41**	**0.7170**	**0.0561**
PD $\rightarrow T_2$	21.46	0.7481	0.0658	**27.43**	**0.9116**	**0.0248**
$T_1 \rightarrow$ MRA	17.80	0.4678	0.1756	**25.03**	**0.7378**	**0.0736**
$T_1 \rightarrow$ PD	19.99	0.6168	0.0834	**21.92**	**0.6869**	**0.0539**
$T_1 \rightarrow T_2$	**19.69**	0.5850	0.0903	19.29	**0.6510**	**0.0615**

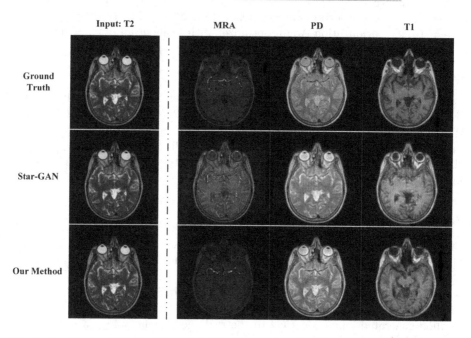

Fig. 2. Synthesis of MRA, PD-weighted and T_1-weighted images using a single T_2-weighted image as input.

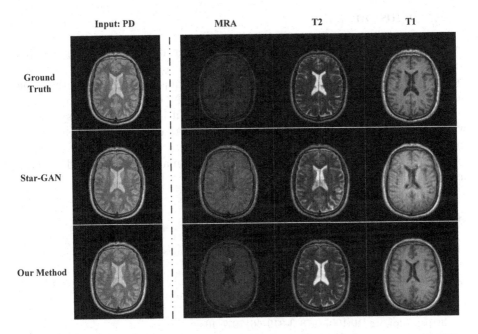

Fig. 3. Synthesis of MRA, T_2-weighted and T_1-weighted images using a single PD-weighted image as input.

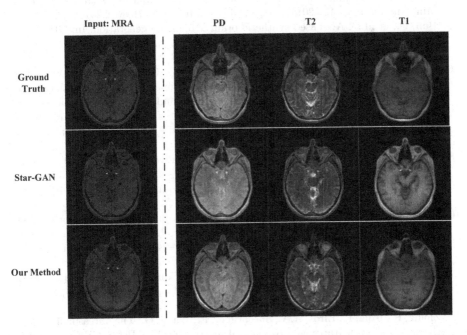

Fig. 4. Synthesis of PD, T_2-weighted and T_1-weighted images using a single MRA image as input.

4 Conclusion

In this paper, we proposed a Star-GAN based method with U-NET generator and new generation loss for multi-contrast MR image synthesis using only one generator and discriminator. The qualitative and quantitative results show the superiority of our method against default Star-GAN. Our solution also removes the limitation of training multiple networks for multi-contrast image synthesis, which is extremely important for many deep learning methods dependent on multi-contrast data for training. In our future work, we would like to extend our experiments to include more modalities and learn mappings among all of them using only a single generator and discriminator.

References

1. Katti, G., Ara, S.A., Shireen, A.: Magnetic resonance imaging (MRI) - a review. Int. J. Dent. Clin. **3**, 65–70 (2011)
2. Joyce, T., Chartsias, A., Tsaftaris, S.A.: Robust Multi-modal MR image synthesis. In: Descoteaux, M., Maier-Hein, L., Franz, A., Jannin, P., Collins, D.L., Duchesne, S. (eds.) MICCAI 2017. LNCS, vol. 10435, pp. 347–355. Springer, Cham (2017). https://doi.org/10.1007/978-3-319-66179-7_40
3. Beers, A., et al.: High-resolution medical image synthesis using progressively grown generative adversarial networks (2018)
4. Liu, J., et al.: Applications of deep learning to MRI images: a survey. Big Data Min. Anal. **1**(1), 1–18 (2018). https://doi.org/10.26599/BDMA.2018.9020001
5. Han, C., et al.: GAN-based synthetic brain MR image generation. In: 2018 IEEE 15th International Symposium on Biomedical Imaging (ISBI 2018), pp. 734–738 (2018). https://doi.org/10.1109/ISBI.2018.8363678
6. Choi, Y., Choi, M., Kim, M., Ha, J.W., Kim, S., Choo, J.: StarGAN: unified generative adversarial networks for multi-domain image-to-image translation. In: 2018 IEEE/CVF Conference on Computer Vision and Pattern Recognition (2018)
7. Zhu, J.Y., Park, T., Isola, P., Efros, A.A.: Unpaired image-to-image translation using cycle-consistent adversarial networks. In: 2017 IEEE International Conference on Computer Vision (ICCV) (2017)
8. Mirza, M., Osindero, S.: Conditional generative adversarial nets. arXiv e-prints arXiv:1411.1784 (2014)
9. Isola, P., Zhu, J.Y., Zhou, T., Efros, A.A.: Image-to-image translation with conditional adversarial networks. In: CVPR (2017)
10. Ronneberger, O., Fischer, P., Brox, T.: U-Net: convolutional networks for biomedical image segmentation. In: Navab, N., Hornegger, J., Wells, W.M., Frangi, A.F. (eds.) MICCAI 2015. LNCS, vol. 9351, pp. 234–241. Springer, Cham (2015). https://doi.org/10.1007/978-3-319-24574-4_28
11. Bovik, A.C., Sheikh, H.R., Simoncelli, E.P.: Image quality assessment: from error visibility to structural similarity. IEEE Trans. Image Process. **13**(4), 600–612 (2004). https://doi.org/10.1109/TIP.2003.819861
12. Zhang, R., Isola, P., Efros, A.A., Shechtman, E., Wang, O.: The unreasonable effectiveness of deep features as a perceptual metric. In: 2018 IEEE/CVF Conference on Computer Vision and Pattern Recognition (2018)

13. Wei, X., Gong, B., Liu, Z., Lu, W., Wang, L.: Improving the improved training of Wasserstein GANs: a consistency term and its dual effect. arXiv e-prints arXiv:1803.01541 (2018)
14. Goodfellow, I.J., et al.: Generative adversarial nets. In: Proceedings of the 27th International Conference on Neural Information Processing Systems, NIPS 2014, vol. 2, pp. 2672–2680. MIT Press, Cambridge (2014). http://dl.acm.org/citation. cfm?id=2969033.2969125
15. Xiang, L., Li, Y., Lin, W., Wang, Q., Shen, D.: Unpaired deep cross-modality synthesis with fast training. In: Stoyanov, D., et al. (eds.) DLMIA/ML-CDS - 2018. LNCS, vol. 11045, pp. 155–164. Springer, Cham (2018). https://doi.org/10. 1007/978-3-030-00889-5_18

Unsupervised Retina Image Synthesis via Disentangled Representation Learning

Kang Li[(✉)], Lequan Yu, Shujun Wang, and Pheng-Ann Heng

The Chinese University of Hong Kong, Hong Kong, China
lk11193875112@gmail.com

Abstract. Fluorescein Fundus Angiography (FFA) is an effective and necessary imaging technology for many retinal diseases including choroiditis, preretinal hemorrhage, and diabetic retinopathy. However, due to the invasive operation, harmful fluorescein dye, and the consequent side effects and complications, it is also an image modality that both doctors and patients are reluctant to use. Therefore, we propose an approach to use Fluorescein Fundus (FF) images, which are non-invasive and safe, to synthesize the invasive and harmful FFA images. Additionally, since paired data are rare and time-consuming to get, the proposed method uses unpaired data to synthesize FFA images in an unsupervised way. Previous unpaired image synthesis methods treat image translation between two domains in two separate ways and thus ignore the implicit feature correlation in the translation process. To solve that, the proposed method first disentangles domain features into domain-shared structure features and domain-independent appearance features. Guided by the adversarial learning, two generators will learn to synthesize FFA-like images and FF-like images correspondingly. Perceptual loss are introduced to preserve the content consistency during translation. Qualitative results show that our model could generate realistic and mimic images without the usage of paired data. We also make quantitative comparisons on Isfahan MISP dataset to demonstrate the superior image quality of the synthetic images.

Keywords: Unsupervised image synthesis · Disentangled representation learning · Fundus images · Fundus angiography images

1 Introduction

Fluorescein Fundus Angiography (FFA) is widely used for imaging the functional state of retinal circulation [13]. With angiographic imaging, detailed information of human retina fundus are enhanced and augmented including vessels and granular structures, which make it a routine diagnostic tool for disease diagnosis including choroiditis, preretinal hemorrhage and diabetic retinopathy [1,14]. However, it is an image modality that both doctors and patients are reluctant to use. Invasive operation, harmful fluorescein dye, consequent side effects and potential complications force physicians only use it in severe situations [10].

© Springer Nature Switzerland AG 2019
N. Burgos et al. (Eds.): SASHIMI 2019, LNCS 11827, pp. 32–41, 2019.
https://doi.org/10.1007/978-3-030-32778-1_4

Moreover, conventional Fluorescein Fundus (FF) imaging is non-invasive and safe. It is a widely used technique for early diagnosis and regular checkup in hospitals. Since the common retina structures like vessels and granular structures are shared in both domains, we propose an approach to use non-invasive and safe FF images to synthesize the invasive and harmful FFA images. Synthesizing FFA images could help doctors to diagnosis with smaller potential risk in patients and relatively reduce the need for actual angiographic imaging.

Medical image synthesis and translation between different domains has been well studied in the past several years. Considering large radiation explosion of CT, Nie et al. [11,12] proposed a context-aware generative adversarial network to synthesize CT images from MRI images. However, their methods need paired data, which are hard to obtain in practice. Chartsias et al. [2] presented an approach based on latent representation, which aims to synthesize multi-output images with multi-input MRI brain images. Similarly, their methods also required aligned image pairs as input. Moreover, their methods focused more about the discovery of modality-invariant content features and ignore the modality-specific features. As image pairs from two image domains of the same patient with the same disease are relatively rare and creates higher demands for data acquisition, the proposed image synthesis method is based on unpaired data in an unsupervised way.

There are also several image synthesis works focused on retina fundus images. Zhao et al. [16,17] and Costa et al. [3] synthesized retina fundus images based on the corresponding segmentation masks for the purpose of data augmentation, segmentation and other usages. These approaches also required fundus images and the corresponding masks to construct training pairs, which similarly also cause difficulty for data acquisition.

Hervella et al. [5] and Schiffers et al. [13] share a similar motivation with us. They also developed approaches to generate FFA images based on retina fundus images. Similar to previous methods, Hervella et al. [5] constructed a Unet architecture with fundus images as input and FFA images as output to learn a direct mapping between two domains. Without the help of adversarial learning, their method leads the model to learn a pixel-to-pixel mapping instead of distribution-to-distribution mapping. Due to the scarcity of paired data, the model would easily become overfitting, which deteriorates the generalization ability of the model.

Schiffers et al. [13] handled this problem with the unpaired data. Inspired by CycleGAN [18], their approach adopted the cycle consistency loss to add reverse mapping for the image translation from FF domain to FFA domain. However, CycleGAN-based methods use two separate generators to learn the translation between two domains, which ignores the implicit relationship of feature translation during the image synthesis process. To be more specific, during translation, structure features are shared in both domains including vessels and granular structure. On the contrary, appearance features are distinctive between two domains like color. As CycleGAN [18] does not utilize these information, the translation process is less controllable.

To solve that, we proposed an unsupervised image synthesis method via disentangled representation learning based on unpaired data. Our approach is based on an assumption that images from two domains could be mapped to the same latent representation in a shared space [8,9]. Inspired by that, we use three encoders to disentangle the domain features into domain-shared structure features and domain-independent appearance features. After that, FFA appearance features are fused with domain-shared structure features to synthesize the required FFA-like images by FFA domain generator. We also put domain-shared structure features into FF domain generator to help stabilize the training process. By adversarial learning, two generators are pushed to synthesize FFA-like images and FF-like images respectively. Moreover, we apply perceptual loss to preserve the structural information during translation. The proposed method is evaluated on public Isfahan MISP dataset [4] with other state-of-the-art methods. Qualitative analysis shows that our methods could generate mimic FFA images. Meanwhile the quantitative comparison demonstrates our method could produce synthetic images with superior image quality over other methods.

2   Methodology

Our method aims to learn a image distribution mapping from domain FF to domain FFA without paired data. To be more specific, for any synthetic FFA image, it should have the structure of the FF image it generates from, combined with the appearance of domain FFA. In the following section, we introduce the disentanglement of domain-shared structure features and domain-independent appearance features first. After that, we describe perceptual loss to make sure the structure-consistency during image translation process. We also introduced other important loss including KL loss and adversarial loss in the end of this section.

2.1   Disentanglement of Structure Features and Appearance Features

There exist common structures like vessels and granular structures between domain FF and domain FFA. Intuitively we use two structure encoders to extract the common features that are shared in two domains $\{E_{FF}^S, E_{FFA}^S\}$. Meanwhile, we use one appearance encoder E_{FFA}^A to capture the independent FFA attributes. Besides that, we also adopt generators $\{G_{FF}, G_{FFA}\}$ and discriminators $\{D_{FF}, D_{FFA}\}$ for two domains, as shown in Fig. 1.

To better deal with non-corresponding data, there are two stages in our model. The forward translation stage learns a mapping from real images to generated images as follows:

$$fake\_FFA = G_{FFA}\left(E_{FFA}^A(I_{FFA}), E_{FF}^S(I_{FF})\right), \tag{1}$$

$$fake\_FF = G_{FF}\left(E_{FFA}^S(I_{FFA})\right). \tag{2}$$

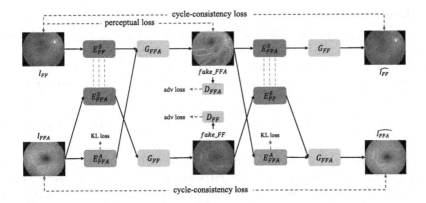

Fig. 1. Model Architecture, where the green and blue blocks represent for structure encoders and appearance encoders. Yellow blocks stand for generators and discriminators. Green dotted lines stand for shared weights between structure encoders. (Color figure online)

Beside that, in backward translation stage, we add a reverse mapping from the generated images back to real images [18], which is formulated as:

$$I_{\hat{F}FA} = G_{FFA}\left(E^A_{FFA}\left(fake\_FFA\right), E^S_{FF}\left(fake\_FF\right)\right), \tag{3}$$

$$I_{\hat{F}F} = G_{FF}\left(E^S_{FFA}\left(fake\_FFA\right)\right). \tag{4}$$

To achieve better representation disentanglement, we apply weight sharing strategy and perceptual loss. For the weight sharing strategy, We let the last layer of E^S_{FF} and E^S_{FFA} to share weights based on the assumption that two domains share one latent content space [9]. The weight sharing strategy could effectively map the domain-shared structure information between two domains into the same latent space.

Moreover, to make sure the generated FFA images could preserve as much as content features of FF images, we construct a perceptual loss between the real FF images and fake FFA images by using the features of a well-trained network. Since a well-trained model contains rich high-level semantic features, it implies that if the real images and generated images have the same structure information, after feeding them into a pre-trained model, they should produce similar high-level features [6,15]. Therefore, the distance of the features above could be act as an evaluation metric of content similarity. Based on that, we construct a perceptual loss to preserve structure-consistency as:

$$\mathcal{L}_p = \|\phi_l\left(I_{FFA}\right) - \phi_l(fake\_FFA)\|_2^2, \tag{5}$$

where $\phi_l(x)$ represents for the $con3, 3$ layer in VGG-19 network [6].

2.2   Loss Functions

Cycle-Consistency Loss. Since there is no paired data involved in the image translation process, we constrain the image translation process by forcing the generated images could be translated back into real images and add L1 loss between the constructed images and input images. The cycle-consistency loss of two domains is defined as:

$$\mathcal{L}_{cc} = \mathbb{E}_{FF \sim p(FF)} \left[\|I_{FF} - \hat{I}_{FF}\|_1 \right] + \mathbb{E}_{FFA \sim p(FFA)} \left[\|I_{FFA} - \hat{I}_{FFA}\|_1 \right]. \quad (6)$$

KL Loss. Since the encoder-generator architecture is basically a Variation Auto-encoder (VAE), we introduce the KL divergence loss in appearance feature extraction. KL loss forces the appearance representation $z_{FFA} = E^A_{FFA}(I_{FFA})$ to be close to the normal Gaussian distribution $p(z) \sim N(0, 1)$, which would help suppress the structure information contained in z_{FFA}. The KL loss is defined as:

$$KL \left(q\left(z_{FFA}\right) \| p(z) \right) = - \int q\left(z_{FFA}\right) \log \frac{p(z)}{q\left(z_{FFA}\right)} dz. \quad (7)$$

In VAE, minimizing KL loss is equivalent to minimizing the following equation [7]:

$$\mathcal{L}_{KL} = \frac{1}{2} \sum_{i=1}^{N} \left(\mu_i^2 + \sigma_i^2 - \log\left(\sigma_i^2\right) - 1 \right), \quad (8)$$

where μ and σ are the mean and standard deviation of appearance feature z_{FFA}. And z_{FFA} is sampled as $z_{FFA} = \mu + z \circ \sigma$, where $\circ$ is the element-wise multiplication.

Adversarial Loss. To generate more realistic and mimic images, we impose domain adversarial loss. The adversarial loss of two domains are formulated as:

$$\mathcal{L}_{D_{FFA}} = \mathbb{E}_{FFA \sim p(FFA)} \left[\log D_{FFA}(I_{FFA}) \right] +$$
$$\mathbb{E}_{FF \sim p(FF)} \left[\log \left(1 - D_{FFA} \left(G_{FFA} \left(E^S_{FF}(I_{FF}), E^A_{FFA}(I_{FF}) \right) \right) \right) \right], \quad (9)$$

$$\mathcal{L}_{D_{FF}} = \mathbb{E}_{FF \sim p(FF)} \left[\log D_{FF}(I_{FF}) \right] +$$
$$\mathbb{E}_{FFA \sim p(FFA)} \left[\log \left(1 - D_{FF} \left(G_{FF} \left(E^S_{FFA}(I_{FFA}) \right) \right) \right) \right]. \quad (10)$$

The generator tries to generate mimic fake images to fool the discriminator, while the discriminator tries to distinguish between the real images and fake images.

The full objective function is formed by the weighted sum of perceptual loss, KL loss, cycle-consistency loss and adversarial loss as follows:

$$\mathcal{L} = \lambda_{adv}\mathcal{L}_{adv} + \lambda_{KL}\mathcal{L}_{KL} + \lambda_{cc}\mathcal{L}_{cc} + \lambda_p\mathcal{L}_p, \quad (11)$$

where $\mathcal{L}_{adv} = \mathcal{L}_{D_{FFA}} + \mathcal{L}_{D_{FF}}$ and the hyper-parameters are setting empirically. In testing, there still needs one FFA image as appearance guide image. According to our observation, the FFA images have minor appearance differences and the choice of guide images has little influence to the generated images, which will be demonstrated in detail at the end of next section.

3 Experiments and Results

3.1 Dataset

In experiments, we use Isfahan MISP dataset which contains 59 image pairs in total [4]. In specific, 30 pairs are healthy cases and 29 pairs are abnormal cases with diabetic retinopathy. We randomly pick 29 pairs as the training set and leave the remaining 30 pairs as the test set. It is worth to mention that the images fed into our methods and Schiffers *et al.* [13] are randomly chosen and randomly cut into patches to make sure no pair information is involved during the training. Also, since our methods needs a FFA image as appearance guide image in testing, the guide image is also randomly picked. The choice of guide images has very little influence to the final results, which will be demonstrated in the end of this section.

3.2 Technique Details

In order to extract more details, we cut the whole images with the resolution of 720×576 into 256×256 patches and perform data augmentation including rotation, random crop and random flip. The structure encoder E^S_{FFA} and E^S_{FF} consist of 3 convolution layers and 4 residual blocks where the last residual block shares weights with each other. For the appearance encoder E^A_{FFA}, we use four convolution layers and one fully connected layer in the end. The generator G_{FFA} and G_{FF} have a symmetric architecture to the structure encoder, which are constructed by 4 residual blocks and 3 transposed convolution layers. In the training process, Adam optimizer is used to update discriminator first and generator and encoder later with beta1 and beta2 setting to 0.5 and 0.999 respectively. The initial learning rate is set to be 0.0001 for the first 50 epochs and linearly decayed for the following 50 epochs. During training, the hyper-parameters λ_{adv}, λ_{cc}, λ_{KL} and λ_{pp} set to be 1, 10, 0.01 and 0.001 respectively. The entire training requires around 6 h computed with one NVIDIA TITAN V GPU card.

3.3 Qualitative Analysis

We compare our results with Hervella *et al.* [5] and Schiffers *et al.* [13], which tackle the same task with us. We visualize several synthetic images generated by the comparison methods and our methods in Fig. 2. All three methods could capture main vessel structures in real FF images. However, the results of Hervella *et al.* [5] have low contrast between the vessels and other tissues. The detailed vessels in the center blend into the surroundings which causes difficulty to observe. Schiffer *et al.* [13] produces better image contrast and highlights the vessels. However, direct mapping between two domains without structure consistency constrain makes the model lack the ability to preserve tiny details like small vessels in the center, which are enlarged and illustrated in Fig. 3 for better image contrast. On the other side, our results preserve the basic vessel structure with clear edges and keep the detailed vessels as well. Moreover, our results have similar appearance to real FFA images.

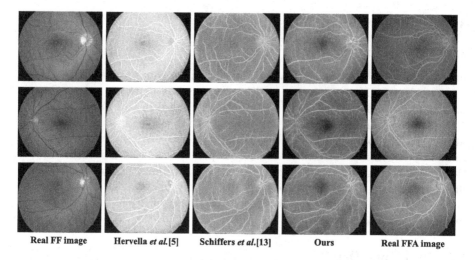

| Real FF image | Hervella *et al.*[5] | Schiffers *et al.*[13] | Ours | Real FFA image |

Fig. 2. Qualitative results of our methods and compared methods.

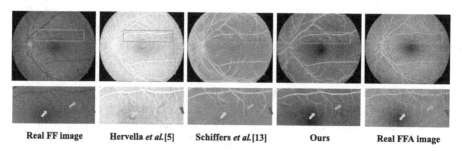

| Real FF image | Hervella *et al.*[5] | Schiffers *et al.*[13] | Ours | Real FFA image |

Fig. 3. Enlarged details of synthetic images generated by our methods and other compared methods, where the first row and second row represent for the original size of synthetic images and the zoom-in details of the red bounding box respectively. The arrows with the same color point out the tiny vessels in the same region. (Color figure online)

3.4   Quantitative Analysis

For quantitative comparison, we use several standard evaluation metrics including Peak signal-to-noise Ratio (PSNR), Mean Squared Error (MSE) and Structural Similarity Index (SSIM) to evaluate the image quality of generated images, as shown in Table 1. Due to the size of training dataset, the method of Hervella *et al.* [5] based on paired data are easy to overfit. Their results are not as good as that of Schiffers *et al.* [13], which utilizes the unpaired images to better exploit feature representation in limited data. The method of Schiffers *et al.* [13] obtains better results in MSE, PSNR and SSIM by 0.0775, 4.7675 and 0.0222 respectively. Meanwhile, as our method takes advantage of domain-shared structure features and domain-independent appearance features in the synthesis process while the approach of Schiffers *et al.* [13] ignores the implicit feature relation-

Table 1. Comparison with other methods in test data.

Methods	MSE ↓	PSNR ↑	SSIM ↑
Hervella *et al.* [5]	0.1181	9.9512	0.5898
Schiffers *et al.* [13]	0.0406	14.7187	0.6312
Ours	0.0242	16.9094	0.6452

Table 2. Quantitative results of different guide images.

	MSE ↓	PSNR ↑	SSIM ↑
std	0.00043	0.00617	0.00015

ship, our results achieve 2.19% and 0.014% improvements in PSNR and SSIM compared to Schiffers *et al.* [13]. The MSE of our results is also lower than that of Schiffers *et al.* [13] by 0.0164%, which demonstrates the effectiveness of our methods and shows the generated images could well preserve structures in FF images.

Since our method needs a FFA image as the appearance guide image to generate mimic FFA images in testing, we also explore the influence of different guide images to the final synthetic images. In this experiment, all FFA images in training dataset are tested here. We compare the standard deviation (std) of MSE, PSNR and SSIM of our synthetic results under different guide images, which are shown in Table 2.

As shown in Table 2, the std of MSE, PSNR and SSIM are relatively small, which implies the image quality of fake FFA images guided by different FFA images have little fluctuation. It also demonstrates that the choice of guide images has minor effects to the generated images.

4   Discussion and Conclusion

Due to the invasive operation and harmful fluorescein dye of Fluorescein Fundus Angiography, we proposed an image synthesis method based on disentangled representation learning to synthesize mimic FFA images from non-invasive and safe Fluorescein Fundus images. Considering data acquisition, the proposed method is designed for unpaired data in unsupervised way. The features of two domains are disentangled into domain-shared structure features and domain-independent appearance features. By adversarial learning, two domain discriminators push generators to synthesize realistic images. To preserve content features during translation, perceptual loss is applied. Both the quantitative comparison and qualitative analysis demonstrate that our methods could generate competitive mimic results with good image quality compared with the state-of-the-art methods.

Acknowledgements. This work was supported by Hong Kong Research Grants Council under General Research Fund (Project No. 14225616) and Hong Kong Innovation and Technology Commission under ITF ITSP Tier 2 Platform Scheme (Project No. ITS/426/17FP).

References

1. Abràmoff, M.D., Garvin, M.K., Sonka, M.: Retinal imaging and image analysis. IEEE Rev. Biomed. Eng. **3**, 169–208 (2010)
2. Chartsias, A., Joyce, T., Giuffrida, M.V., Tsaftaris, S.A.: Multimodal MR synthesis via modality-invariant latent representation. IEEE Trans. Med. Imaging **37**(3), 803–814 (2018)
3. Costa, P., et al.: End-to-end adversarial retinal image synthesis. IEEE Trans. Med. Imaging **37**(3), 781–791 (2018)
4. Mohammad Alipour, S.H., Rabbani, H., Akhlaghi, M.R.: Diabetic retinopathy grading by digital curvelet transform. Comput. Math. Methods Med. **2012**, 1–11 (2012)
5. Hervella, Á.S., Rouco, J., Novo, J., Ortega, M.: Retinal image understanding emerges from self-supervised multimodal reconstruction. In: Frangi, A.F., Schnabel, J.A., Davatzikos, C., Alberola-López, C., Fichtinger, G. (eds.) MICCAI 2018. LNCS, vol. 11070, pp. 321–328. Springer, Cham (2018). https://doi.org/10.1007/978-3-030-00928-1_37
6. Johnson, J., Alahi, A., Fei-Fei, L.: Perceptual losses for real-time style transfer and super-resolution. In: Leibe, B., Matas, J., Sebe, N., Welling, M. (eds.) ECCV 2016. LNCS, vol. 9906, pp. 694–711. Springer, Cham (2016). https://doi.org/10.1007/978-3-319-46475-6_43
7. Kingma, D.P., Welling, M.: Auto-encoding variational Bayes. arXiv preprint arXiv:1312.6114 (2013)
8. Lee, H.-Y., Tseng, H.-Y., Huang, J.-B., Singh, M., Yang, M.-H.: Diverse image-to-image translation via disentangled representations. In: Ferrari, V., Hebert, M., Sminchisescu, C., Weiss, Y. (eds.) ECCV 2018. LNCS, vol. 11205, pp. 36–52. Springer, Cham (2018). https://doi.org/10.1007/978-3-030-01246-5_3
9. Liu, M.Y., Breuel, T., Kautz, J.: Unsupervised image-to-image translation networks. In: Advances in Neural Information Processing Systems, pp. 700–708 (2017)
10. Musa, F., Muen, W.J., Hancock, R., Clark, D.: Adverse effects of fluorescein angiography in hypertensive and elderly patients. Acta Ophthalmol. Scand. **84**(6), 740–742 (2006)
11. Nie, D., et al.: Medical image synthesis with context-aware generative adversarial networks. In: Descoteaux, M., Maier-Hein, L., Franz, A., Jannin, P., Collins, D.L., Duchesne, S. (eds.) MICCAI 2017. LNCS, vol. 10435, pp. 417–425. Springer, Cham (2017). https://doi.org/10.1007/978-3-319-66179-7_48
12. Nie, D., et al.: Medical image synthesis with deep convolutional adversarial networks. IEEE Trans. Biomed. Eng. **65**(12), 2720–2730 (2018)
13. Schiffers, F., Yu, Z., Arguin, S., Maier, A., Ren, Q.: Synthetic fundus fluorescein angiography using deep neural networks. Bildverarbeitung für die Medizin 2018. I, pp. 234–238. Springer, Heidelberg (2018). https://doi.org/10.1007/978-3-662-56537-7_64
14. Shoughy, S.S., Kozak, I.: Selective and complementary use of optical coherence tomography and fluorescein angiography in retinal practice. Eye Vis. **3**(1), 26 (2016)

15. Taigman, Y., Polyak, A., Wolf, L.: Unsupervised cross-domain image generation. arXiv preprint arXiv:1611.02200 (2016)
16. Zhao, H., Li, H., Maurer-Stroh, S., Cheng, L.: Synthesizing retinal and neuronal images with generative adversarial nets. Med. Image Anal. **49**, 14–26 (2018)
17. Zhao, H., Li, H., Maurer-Stroh, S., Guo, Y., Deng, Q., Cheng, L.: Supervised segmentation of un-annotated retinal fundus images by synthesis. IEEE Trans. Med. Imaging **38**(1), 46–56 (2019)
18. Zhu, J.Y., Park, T., Isola, P., Efros, A.A.: Unpaired image-to-image translation using cycle-consistent adversarial networks. In: Proceedings of the IEEE International Conference on Computer Vision, pp. 2223–2232 (2017)

Pseudo-normal PET Synthesis with Generative Adversarial Networks for Localising Hypometabolism in Epilepsies

Siti Nurbaya Yaakub[1,2]([✉]), Colm J. McGinnity[1,2], James R. Clough[1], Eric Kerfoot[1], Nadine Girard[3], Eric Guedj[4,5], and Alexander Hammers[1,2]

[1] School of Biomedical Engineering & Imaging Sciences, King's College London, London, UK
siti_nurbaya.yaakub@kcl.ac.uk
[2] King's College London & GSTT PET Centre, St. Thomas' Hospital, London, UK
[3] Neuroradiology Department, Assistance Publique Hôpitaux de Marseille, Marseille, France
[4] Nuclear Medicine Department, Assistance Publique Hôpitaux de Marseille, Marseille, France
[5] Institut Fresnel, Aix-Marseille Universitè, CNRS, Ecole Centrale Marseille, Marseille, France

Abstract. [^{18}F]fluorodeoxyglucose (FDG) positron emission tomography (PET) aids in the localisation of the epileptogenic zone in patients with focal epilepsy, especially when magnetic resonance imaging (MRI) is normal or non-contributory. We propose a two-stage deep learning framework to support the clinical evaluation of patients with focal epilepsy by identifying candidate regions of hypometabolism in [^{18}F]FDG PET scans. In the first stage, we train a generative adversarial network (GAN) to learn the mapping between healthy [^{18}F]FDG PET and T1-weighted (T1w) MRI data. In the second stage, we synthesise pseudo-normal PET images from T1w MRI scans of patients with epilepsy to compare to the real PET scans. Comparing the estimated pseudo-PET images to the true PET scans in healthy control data, our GAN produced whole-brain mean absolute errors of 0.053 ± 0.015, outperforming a U-Net (0.058 ± 0.021) and a high-resolution dilated convolutional neural network (0.060 ± 0.024; all images scaled 0–1). In a sample of 20 epilepsy patients, we created Z-statistic images (with thresholding at $+2.33$) by subtracting the patient's true PET scans from their estimated pseudo-normal PET images to identify regions of hypometabolism. Excellent sensitivity for lobar location of abnormalities ($92.9 \pm 13.1\%$) was observed for the seven cases with MR-visible epileptogenic lesions. For the 13 cases with non-contributory MR, a lower sensitivity of $74.8 \pm 32.3\%$ was observed. Our method performed better than a statistical parametric mapping analysis. Our results highlight the potential of deep learning-based pseudo-normal [^{18}F]FDG PET synthesis to contribute to the management of epilepsy.

Keywords: PET · MRI · Clinical decision support · Epilepsy · GAN

© Springer Nature Switzerland AG 2019
N. Burgos et al. (Eds.): SASHIMI 2019, LNCS 11827, pp. 42–51, 2019.
https://doi.org/10.1007/978-3-030-32778-1_5

1   Introduction

The accurate localisation of the epileptogenic zone, i.e. the part of the brain that initiates the seizure, is a prerequisite to the surgical management of patients with drug-resistant (i.e. 'refractory') focal epilepsy. This can be extremely challenging, in particular in those with small epileptogenic lesions such as focal cortical dysplasias (FCDs) which are often overlooked (e.g. 33% in [1]) or impossible to visualise on conventional magnetic resonance imaging (MRI) scans (e.g. 28% of patients in [2]). [18F]fluorodeoxyglucose (FDG) positron emission tomography (PET) is used clinically to detect focal reductions of glucose metabolism (hypometabolism) that are characteristic of the epileptogenic zone. Clinical evaluation, which relies on subjective visual analysis and is often performed in the absence of co-registered MRI images, can be challenging and time-consuming even for experts.

Regarding the identification of subtle FCDs, the majority of work to date has neglected the high sensitivity of expertly read co-registered PET, whereas the multi-modal approaches have required time-consuming feature extraction [3]. There are very little data available for research use that have been validated by post-surgical follow-up, and particularly few true MRI-negative cases. Other work has focused on mass univariate approaches in comparison to healthy controls with normalisation to a standard brain template [4].

Recently, T1-weighted (T1w) MRI images have been used to synthesise missing [18F]FDG PET images via 3D convolutional neural networks (CNN) [5], U-Net networks [6], and cycle-consistent generative adversarial networks (GAN) [7]. These methods went on to classify patients with Alzheimer's Disease where hypometabolism is spatially extensive. Pseudo-PET synthesis has so far not been applied to the more challenging problem of detecting small lesions in epilepsy.

The current work aims to use a CNN to synthesise pseudo-normal PET scans from T1w MRIs for the identification of candidate regions of hypometabolism to complement the visual analysis of PET scans in patients with focal epilepsy.

2   Methods

Our method (Fig. 1) consists of two stages. In stage 1, we train a 3D GAN to learn the mapping between T1w MRIs and [18F]FDG PET scans in healthy control data. In stage 2, we use this network to synthesise pseudo-normal [18F]FDG PET scans in patients with epilepsy, based on the patient's T1w MRI. We subtract the patient's real PET scan from the estimated (i.e. synthesised) pseudo-normal PET scan in order to locate areas of hypometabolism.

2.1   Stage 1: Network Architecture

The architecture of our 3D patch GAN model (Fig. 1) is based on [8]. The generator is based on a residual U-Net CNN [9,10], consisting of blocks of two $3 \times 3 \times 3$

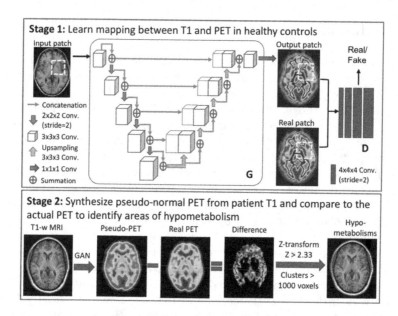

Fig. 1. Two stage method for identifying hypometabolism in patients with epilepsy. Stage 1: 3D patch GAN architecture for estimating pseudo-normal PET from MRI. G: Generator. D: Discriminator. Stage 2: Identifying hypometabolic clusters in patients.

convolutions, each followed by a batch normalisation [11] and PReLU [12] activation. It takes a T1w MRI image patch as input. In the encoding path, instead of max pooling, downsampling is performed using convolutions with a stride of 2. In the decoding path, the upsampled input is concatenated with the output from the encoding path on the same level. The final convolution in the last layer uses a sigmoid activation to output the voxel-wise predictions of PET intensities for the patch. The discriminator consists of five layers of convolution, batch normalisation and PReLU sequences with downsampling using a stride of 2, with 64, 128, 256, 512, and 1 channels each. The input is a pair of real and synthetic PET image patches and the output is a binary real or fake prediction.

We compare our method to a U-Net with the same architecture as the generator in [8]. Since U-Net models have been shown to produce smoother output, we also compare our method to a high-resolution 3D CNN with dilated convolutions [13], which is able to retain high-resolution features across the network without down- or up-sampling. For the dilated CNN, we use the network architecture as described in the original work, with the exception of the final layer, where we replace the softmax with a sigmoid activation.

We use the bias-field corrected T1w MRIs as input and the [18F]FDG PET scans as output. We evaluate the performance of each network by comparing the errors between the network output and ground truth PET images.

2.2   Stage 2: Identification of Hypometabolic Regions

Hypometabolic regions were identified by subtracting each patient's ground truth ('real') PET scan from the estimated pseudo-normal PET scan, converting the values to a Z-score ($Z = (X - \mu) \div \sigma$), where X is the difference value at each voxel, μ is the mean and σ is the standard deviation across the whole image, and thresholding at $Z = 2.33$ (equivalent to a p-value of 0.01). This is similar to the method used in comparing ictal SPECT scans to identify regions of hyperperfusion for epilepsy localisation [14]. Additionally we applied a cluster size threshold of $1000\,\text{mm}^3$, aligned to typical FCD size [15]. We limited the calculation of Z-score within a brain mask generated using FSL BET [16], which was eroded by 3 voxels to give a conservative brain mask.

We compare our method to a mass univariate single subject analysis performed within the statistical parametric mapping (SPM) framework implemented in Matlab using the SPM12 software (fil.ion.ucl.ac.uk/spm). All patient and healthy control PET images were first normalised to MNI space ($2^3\,\text{mm}^3$ spatial resolution). For each patient, a general linear model (GLM) was then fitted to each voxel, with group as the variable of interest. Post-hoc inference on the contrast of interest (controls > patient) was done using a standard mass univariate statistical test resulting in a T-statistic map for each patient. Areas of hypometabolism were identified as clusters of voxels above an uncorrected statistical threshold of $p < 0.001$ with a cluster-forming threshold of $1000\,\text{mm}^3$.

3   Experiments and Results

3.1   PET Synthesis from T1 in Healthy Control Data

Materials. Our training data set consisted of 55 healthy control participants aged between 21 and 78 years (mean age = 49.6 ± 16.2; 32 female) from a database of [18F]FDG PET and MRI scans. The images included a 3D T1w MPRAGE (Siemens MAGNETOM Symphony 1.5T, voxel size = $1\,\text{mm}^3$ matrix size = $160 \times 256 \times 256$) and a 15-minute averaged [18F]FDG PET image (GE Discovery ST PET/CT system, voxel size = $0.8\,\text{mm}^3$, matrix size = $256 \times 256 \times 47$, resampled to 256^3). The PET scan was performed after a bolus intravenous injection of 150 MBq of [18F]FDG and 30-minutes of eyes-closed uptake time. Each participant's PET scan was rigidly aligned to their MRI using NiftyReg [17] and all images were scaled between 0 and 1 and cropped to have a 17 cm cranio-caudal extent to exclude the neck.

Network Training and Cross-Validation of PET Synthesis. We implemented all three network architectures using the Keras framework with the TensorFlow backend on an NVIDIA Quadro M4000 GPU with 8 GB of RAM. Networks were trained on mini-batches of patches each of size $32 \times 32 \times 32$. We used the Adam optimiser with Nesterov momentum [18] and mean squared error (MSE) as the loss, with weights initialised as in [12]. All networks were trained

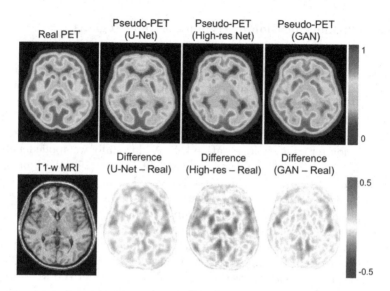

Fig. 2. Examples of synthesised pseudo-normal [^{18}F]FDG PET scans of one healthy control subject. Top, left to right: real PET, synthesised pseudo-PET using the U-Net, high-resolution dilated CNN, and our proposed GAN. Bottom, left to right: T1w MRI, difference maps between synthesised and real PET scans for the U-Net, high-resolution dilated CNN and our proposed GAN. Positive differences indicate higher intensities in the synthesised scan.

with an initial learning rate of 0.0002. The residual U-Net was trained on 25000 mini-batches of 24 patches, the high-resolution CNN was trained on 25000 mini-batches of 8 patches, and the GAN was trained on 10000 mini-batches of 24 patches. We performed a five-fold cross-validation with each fold consisting of 40 training, 4 validation and 11 test cases.

Performance of PET Synthesis Model. We evaluated the performance of the network by comparing the estimated and ground truth PET images using two metrics: the mean absolute error (MAE) and the peak signal-to-noise ratio (PSNR). We compared the MAE and PSNR of PET images synthesised by the GAN to each of the other two methods using paired t-tests. The proposed 3D

Table 1. Performance of PET synthesis models. Mean absolute error (MAE) and peak signal-to-noise ratio (PSNR) are given as mean ± SD across the 5-fold cross-validation.

Model	MAE	PSNR
U-Net	0.058 ± 0.021	22.9 ± 2.6
High-res Net	0.060 ± 0.024	22.8 ± 2.6
GAN	$\mathbf{0.053 \pm 0.015}$	$\mathbf{23.2 \pm 2.3}$

conditional GAN method had significantly lower MAE and higher PSNR values (all $p < 0.05$) compared to each of the other two methods for the 5-fold cross-validation on healthy controls (Table 1). Examples of synthesised pseudo-PETs are shown in (Fig. 2).

3.2 Identification of Hypometabolism in Epilepsy Patients

Materials. We studied 20 patients with drug-resistant epilepsy who were referred for a PET scan as part of their clinical evaluation (age range = 13–70 years; mean age = 32.4 ± 17.3; 13 female). Data was acquired on a whole-body GE Discovery 710 PET/CT system and a 3T Siemens Biograph mMR PET-MR system on the same day. Scans included a 15-minute [^{18}F]FDG PET scan on the PET/CT system 30 min post-injection, and a 3D T1w MPRAGE scan on the PET-MR system (acquired in sagittal orientation, 1.1 mm^3 voxels, $176 \times 224 \times 256$ matrix). MRI scans were bias-field corrected using the N4 algorithm [19] and resampled to 1 mm^3 voxels. Each patient's PET scan was converted to standardised uptake values (SUVs) and linearly aligned to their MRI scan using NiftyReg [17], scaled between 0 and 1, and cropped as above.

All participants provided written informed consent and procedures performed were in accordance with the ethical standards of the Health Research Authority UK National Research Ethics Service (North East – York Research Ethics Committee, approval number: 15/NE/0203).

Validation of Method in Epilepsy Patients. The patients' PET/CT scans were reported by two Consultant Nuclear Medicine Physicians as part of their clinical management. In this proof-of-concept study, we only used patient data where the PET showed abnormalities on visual inspection in order to have ground truth for comparison. Patients were classified as either MRI-positive (n = 7, where both MRI and PET showed abnormalities on visual inspection) or MRI-negative (n = 13, where MRI was normal or non-contributory and PET showed abnormalities).

We trained the GAN on the full database of healthy controls and synthesised a pseudo-normal PET image from the T1w MRI scan of each epilepsy patient, which we compared to the patient's ground truth PET scan. Sensitivity and precision were calculated as compared to the physician's reports. For each cluster of identified hypometabolism, we counted a true positive (TP) if the cluster matched the location described in the patient's clinical PET reading at the lobar level, a false positive (FP) if the cluster was not reported, and a false negative (FN) if no cluster was found where the report described a region of hypometabolism. For each patient, we quantified the sensitivity, or true positive rate $(TP \div (TP + FN))$, and precision, or positive predictive value $(TP \div (TP + FP))$, of the method for detecting hypometabolism.

Table 2. Performance of our method compared to the SPM analysis for hypometabolism detection. Sensitivity and Precision are given as percent mean ± SD. FP and FN refer to False Positive and False Negative clusters respectively.

Method	Sensitivity (%)	Precision (%)	Number of FP	Number of FN
All patients (n = 20)				
Proposed Method	81.1 ± 28.5	52.2 ± 24.5	3.0 ± 1.6	0.8 ± 1.1
SPM Analysis	41.7 ± 46.0	34.0 ± 36.5	1.6 ± 1.7	1.9 ± 2.2
MRI-positive patients (n = 7)				
Proposed Method	92.9 ± 13.1	52.1 ± 11.6	2.6 ± 1.0	0.3 ± 0.5
SPM Analysis	42.9 ± 42.6	52.4 ± 41.3	0.8 ± 0.4	2.6 ± 2.3
MRI-negative patients (n = 13)				
Proposed Method	74.8 ± 32.3	50.7 ± 27.5	3.2 ± 1.8	1.1 ± 1.3
SPM Analysis	41.0 ± 48.7	24.0 ± 30.3	2.0 ± 1.9	1.6 ± 2.2

Performance of Method for Hypometabolism Detection. Results for hypometabolism detection for our proposed method compared to the SPM analysis are shown in Table 2. In 11 of the 20 cases, we had 100% sensitivity, i.e. we were able to identify all the regions of hypometabolism found in the physician's PET reports. We show two example cases of the clusters of hypometabolism detected using our method in Fig. 3.

4   Discussion and Conclusion

We present a two-stage framework utilising deep learning applied to the novel application of detecting hypometabolism in patients with drug-resistant focal epilepsy. In the first stage, we used a GAN to synthesise pseudo-normal [18F]FDG PET images from T1w MRI scans. We found that our GAN significantly outperformed two CNNs, and the MAEs and PSNRs obtained were comparable to previous PET synthesis studies [5, 6]. In the second stage, we subtracted real patient [18F]FDG PET scans from synthesised pseudo-normal [18F]FDG PET images in order to detect clusters of significant hypometabolism. Our method was able to detect hypometabolic regions with high sensitivity in both MRI-positive (93% sensitivity) and MRI-negative (75% sensitivity) patients.

We compared three networks for PET image synthesis from MRI. The U-Net, although traditionally used for image segmentation, has been shown to work well for MRI to PET image synthesis [6], but fails to capture high-resolution detail and produces blurry images. A CNN which is able to maintain high-resolution image features across the network, such as the high-resolution dilated convolutional network, might theoretically work better. However, we found the two CNNs did not differ significantly in terms of the images produced, and the GAN outperformed both methods. This might be because the GAN is more suited to image synthesis. The discriminator loss could potentially pick up on

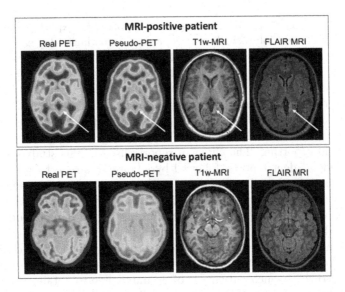

Fig. 3. Examples of hypometabolic clusters detected in an MRI-positive (top) and an MRI-negative (bottom) patient. Left to right: Real [18F]FDG PET scan; synthesised pseudo-normal [18F]FDG PET scan; T1w MRI with clusters of hypometabolism overlaid; T2-FLAIR MRI. We show the patient's T2-FLAIR MRI to highlight the hypometabolism corresponding to the FCD for the MRI-positive case (white arrows).

subtle textural details in a more nuanced way compared to MSE, where the differences between image patches are averaged across the whole patch and hence the shape of the predicted image contributes more to the loss value.

Our method exploits the mismatch between an apparently normal [18F]FDG PET image synthesised from the patient's largely normal T1w MRI, and the patient's actual abnormal [18F]FDG PET scan. It is thus able to provide a "personalised" pseudo-normal template of the patient's [18F]FDG PET uptake, compared to conventional methods (e.g. an SPM-type analysis) where comparison is made via a normalised brain template. Here, we were able to show that our method performs significantly better than a standard SPM analysis. Our method also generalises well to different MR and PET acquisitions as the network was trained on healthy control data obtained from a different site and applied to unseen patient data.

We found higher sensitivity in patients who were MRI-positive than MRI-negative. This could be due to smaller overall numbers in the MRI-positive group. The MRI-positive cases in this study were predominantly temporal lobe lesional cases (5 of 7 cases), and PET is known to be more sensitive than MRI in lesional than in non-lesional temporal lobe epilepsy cases [20]. This might explain the larger mismatch between the pseudo-normal and real PET images, and thus higher sensitivity, in the MRI-positive patients reported here.

While our method does yield roughly 3 false positives per patient, for eight of the 20 patients these clusters were in spatially plausible regions, either in close spatial proximity to the true positive region(s) reported by expert visual analysis, or in the contralateral lobe which may represent secondarily decreased synaptic activity in areas that are connected via commissural fibres. Another explanation may be that less conspicuous abnormalities were not reported. Finally, focal epilepsy is also increasingly appreciated as a network disorder and abnormalities distant from the epileptogenic zone are seen on PET and MRI [21].

We envision the method forming the basis of a tool that could highlight regions of potential clinical significance to the physician, to facilitate comprehensive clinical reporting. The clinician reports used in this study consisted of two initial independent reports, followed by a consensus report after discussion of any mismatch in the reports. Future work to assess the effectiveness of the method as a complementary tool could involve a further tertiary review of the PET images with the help of the clusters obtained from our method, however this is beyond the scope of the present paper.

We were unable to evaluate the method in the most challenging clinical subpopulation, i.e. MR- and PET-negative patients. This limitation is common as the "ground truth" in such patients is often impossible to obtain. Post-surgical follow-up of the cases described herein, as well as validation in a larger patient population has the potential to build confidence in the method in general. Further studies will allow the optimisation of the cluster-forming thresholds through receiver operating characteristic curves across a range of thresholds.

In conclusion, our results demonstrate that the proposed two-stage approach yields accurate pseudo-normal PET images and has potential clinical value as an objective complement to expert visual analyses.

References

1. Kreilkamp, B., Das, K., Wieshmann, U., Biswas, S., Marson, A., Keller, S.: Neuroradiological findings in patients with "non-lesional" focal epilepsy revealed by research protocol. Clin. Radiol. **74**(1), 78.e1–78.e11 (2019). https://doi.org/10.1016/j.crad.2018.08.013
2. Widdess-Walsh, P., et al.: Electro-clinical and imaging characteristics of focal cortical dysplasia: correlation with pathological subtypes. Epilepsy Res. **67**(1–2), 25–33 (2005). https://doi.org/10.1016/j.eplepsyres.2005.07.013
3. Tan, Y.L., et al.: Quantitative surface analysis of combined MRI and PET enhances detection of focal cortical dysplasias. NeuroImage **166**, 10–18 (2018). https://doi.org/10.1016/j.neuroimage.2017.10.065
4. Zhu, Y., et al.: Glucose metabolic profile by visual assessment combined with statistical parametric mapping analysis in pediatric patients with epilepsy. J. Nucl. Med. **58**(8), 1293–1299 (2017). https://doi.org/10.2967/jnumed.116.187492
5. Li, R., et al.: Deep learning based imaging data completion for improved brain disease diagnosis. In: Golland, P., Hata, N., Barillot, C., Hornegger, J., Howe, R. (eds.) MICCAI 2014. LNCS, vol. 8675, pp. 305–312. Springer, Cham (2014). https://doi.org/10.1007/978-3-319-10443-0_39
6. Sikka, A., Peri, S.V., Bathula, D.R.: MRI to FDG-PET: cross-modal synthesis using 3D U-Net for multi-modal Alzheimer's classification. In: Gooya, A., Goksel, O., Oguz, I., Burgos, N. (eds.) SASHIMI 2018. LNCS, vol. 11037, pp. 80–89. Springer, Cham (2018). https://doi.org/10.1007/978-3-030-00536-8_9

7. Pan, Y., Liu, M., Lian, C., Zhou, T., Xia, Y., Shen, D.: Synthesizing missing PET from MRI with cycle-consistent generative adversarial networks for Alzheimer's disease diagnosis. In: Frangi, A.F., Schnabel, J.A., Davatzikos, C., Alberola-López, C., Fichtinger, G. (eds.) MICCAI 2018. LNCS, vol. 11072, pp. 455–463. Springer, Cham (2018). https://doi.org/10.1007/978-3-030-00931-1_52

8. Isola, P., Zhu, J.Y., Zhou, T., Efros, A.A.: Image-to-image translation with conditional adversarial networks. In: CVPR 2017, pp. 5967–5976. IEEE (2017). https://doi.org/10.1109/CVPR.2017.632

9. Ronneberger, O., Fischer, P., Brox, T.: U-Net: convolutional networks for biomedical image segmentation. In: Navab, N., Hornegger, J., Wells, W.M., Frangi, A.F. (eds.) MICCAI 2015. LNCS, vol. 9351, pp. 234–241. Springer, Cham (2015). https://doi.org/10.1007/978-3-319-24574-4_28

10. He, K., Zhang, X., Ren, S., Sun, J.: Deep residual learning for image recognition. In: CVPR 2016, pp. 770–778. IEEE (2016). https://doi.org/10.1109/CVPR.2016.90

11. Ioffe, S., Szegedy, C.: Batch normalization: accelerating deep network training by reducing internal covariate shift. In: Bach, F., Blei, D. (eds.) ICML 2015, vol. 37, pp. 448–456. PMLR, Lille (2015)

12. He, K., Zhang, X., Ren, S., Sun, J.: Delving deep into rectifiers: surpassing human-level performance on ImageNet classification. In: ICCV 2015, pp. 1026–1034. IEEE (2015). https://doi.org/10.1109/ICCV.2015.123

13. Li, W., Wang, G., Fidon, L., Ourselin, S., Cardoso, M.J., Vercauteren, T.: On the compactness, efficiency, and representation of 3D convolutional networks: brain parcellation as a pretext task. In: Niethammer, M., et al. (eds.) IPMI 2017. LNCS, vol. 10265, pp. 348–360. Springer, Cham (2017). https://doi.org/10.1007/978-3-319-59050-9_28

14. O'Brien, T.J., et al.: Subtraction ictal SPECT co-registered to MRI improves clinical usefulness of SPECT in localizing the surgical seizure focus. Nucl. Med. Commun. **19**, 31–45 (1998)

15. Colliot, O., Antel, S.B., Naessens, V.B., Bernasconi, N., Bernasconi, A.: In vivo profiling of focal cortical dysplasia on high-resolution MRI with computational models. Epilepsia **47**(1), 134–142 (2006). https://doi.org/10.1111/j.1528-1167.2006.00379.x

16. Smith, S.M.: Fast robust automated brain extraction. Hum. Brain Mapp. **17**(3), 143–155 (2002). https://doi.org/10.1002/hbm.10062

17. Modat, M., et al.: Fast free-form deformation using graphics processing units. Comput. Methods Programs Biomed. **98**(3), 278–284 (2010). https://doi.org/10.1016/j.cmpb.2009.09.002

18. Sutskever, I., Martens, J., Dahl, G., Hinton, G.: On the importance of initialization and momentum in deep learning. In: Dasgupta, S., McAllester, D. (eds.) ICML 2013, vol. 28, pp. 1139–1147. PMLR (2013)

19. Tustison, N.J., et al.: N4ITK: improved N3 bias correction. IEEE Trans. Med. Imaging **29**(6), 1310–1320 (2010). https://doi.org/10.1109/TMI.2010.2046908

20. Spencer, S.S., Theodore, W.H., Berkovic, S.F.: Clinical applications: MRI, SPECT, and PET. Magn. Reson. Imaging **13**(8), 1119–1124 (1995). https://doi.org/10.1016/0730-725X(95)02021-K

21. Kramer, M.A., Cash, S.S.: Epilepsy as a disorder of cortical network organization. Neuroscientist **18**(4), 360–372 (2012). https://doi.org/10.1177/1073858411422754

Breast Mass Detection in Mammograms via Blending Adversarial Learning

Chunze Lin[1], Ruixiang Tang[1], Darryl D. Lin[2], Langechuan Liu[2], Jiwen Lu[1(✉)], Yunqiang Chen[2], Dashan Gao[2], and Jie Zhou[1]

[1] Tsinghua University, Beijing, China
{lcz16,trx14}@mails.tsinghua.edu.cn,
{lujiwen,jzhou}@tsinghua.edu.cn
[2] 12 Sigma Technologies, San Diego, USA
{dlin,pliu,yunqiang,dgao}@12sigma.ai

Abstract. Deep learning approaches have recently been proposed for breast cancer screening in mammograms. However, the performance of such deep models is often severely constrained by the limited size of publicly available mammography datasets and the imbalance of healthy and abnormal images. In this paper, we propose a blending adversarial learning method to address this issue by regularizing the imbalanced data with synthetically generated abnormal samples. Unlike most existing data generation methods that require large-scale training data, our approach is carefully designed for augmenting small datasets. Specifically, we train a generative model to simulate the growth of mass on normal tissue by blending mass patches into healthy breast images. The resulting synthetic images are exploited as complementary abnormal data to make the training of deep learning based mass detector more stable and the resulting model more robust. Experimental results on the commonly used INbreast dataset demonstrate the effectiveness of the proposed method.

Keywords: Mammogram synthesis · Mass detection · Adversarial deep learning · Digital mammography

1 Introduction

Breast cancer is among the most common cancers affecting women around the world. Mammography has been demonstrated to be an effective imaging modality for early detection and diagnosis, and has contributed to substantial reduction of mortality due to breast cancer. Over the past few years, computer-aided detection of breast masses in mammography has attracted much attention from the medical imaging community [1,3,8,9,15].

Recently, with the prevalent success of deep learning in natural image applications, there has been keen interest in the medical imaging community to apply these methods to mammogram screening. However, deep convolutional neural networks (CNN) based approaches require a large amount of annotated data.

© Springer Nature Switzerland AG 2019
N. Burgos et al. (Eds.): SASHIMI 2019, LNCS 11827, pp. 52–61, 2019.
https://doi.org/10.1007/978-3-030-32778-1_6

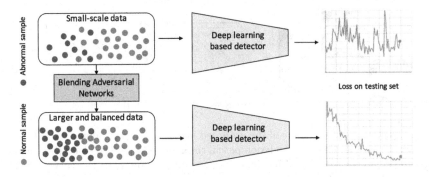

Fig. 1. Training a detector with small-scale and imbalanced datasets leads to unsatisfactory results. Our blending adversarial networks help to increase the scale of the datasets and address the class imbalance issues for training more robust detector.

The lack of such data has become the main obstacle impeding deep learning methods from achieving impressive performance for breast cancer screening. In contrast to the natural image domain, collecting annotated breast mammograms is very expensive due to the need for expert annotation and oftentimes difficult or even impossible because of privacy restrictions. In addition to the lack of large-scale datasets, the natural class imbalance in mammography samples, where "normal" (or healthy) images significantly outnumber abnormal samples, further limits the performance of deep CNN based methods for breast cancer detection, as illustrated in Fig. 1.

A common way to alleviate these issues involves applying a series of transformations such as flipping, rotation or resizing to augment the training images. However, data augmentation using image transformation is limited in its ability to expand the manifold the positive samples occupy. More recently, generative adversarial networks (GANs) [4] have demonstrated the capability to synthesize realistic images that can be used for data augmentation. For example, Korkinof *et al.* [9] utilized the progressive generative adversarial network to generate high resolution mammograms. Wu *et al.* [15] proposed the conditional infilling GANs to generate lesions on non-malignant patches. One major drawback of these methods is that they rely on a large amount of data to train the generator, making them unsuitable for small-scale datasets.

In this paper, we propose blending adversarial networks to address the limitation of small-scale and imbalanced data for mass detection in mammogram. GANs based methods usually train a generator to synthesize mammograms from Gaussian distributed random values. This demands the generator to learn the texture, the shape and the size of the breast and lesion. Learning to synthesize these features requires inevitably a large-scale training dataset. As opposed to such a heavy task, we simplify the burden of the generator: we provide both the real lesion and "normal" image at the input, and train a model to imagine how this lesion will grow on the normal breast tissue. Since the information about the lesion and breast are given, the generator can focus on integrating the lesion

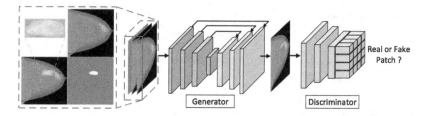

Fig. 2. Overview of the pipeline of the proposed blending adversarial networks. Given a real "normal" breast image and a lesion patch, the generator aims to blend these images at the indicated location. The discriminator verifies the quality of the generated data at patch level forcing the generator to produce highly realistic images.

into healthy breast tissue. By simplifying the task of the generator, we can train it even with a very small dataset. Therefore, we are able to utilize "normal" images to artificially generate abnormal mammograms to increase the data size and alleviate class imbalance. Extensive experiments on widely-used INbreast dataset [11] demonstrate the effectiveness of the proposed method, where the mass detector becomes significantly more robust when trained with the complementary synthetic samples.

2   Methodology

Mathematically, given a set of "normal" images $\mathbf{X} = \{X_1, ..., X_N\}$ and a set of lesion patches $\mathbf{E} = \{E_1, ..., E_M\}$, our goal is to learn a network to seamlessly blend the lesions into the "normal" images to form a new set of images containing lesions $\tilde{\mathbf{Y}} = \{\tilde{Y}_1, ..., \tilde{Y}_L\}$. The proposed blending adversarial networks can be learned from a small-scale dataset to generate new images. We then include them as the complementary training samples to train a deep learning based breast mass detector, making it more robust and effective.

2.1   Blending Adversarial Networks

In Fig. 2, we illustrate the pipeline of our blending adversarial networks, composing mainly of a generator and a patch discriminator. Unlike the vanilla GANs [4] which rely on large-scale datasets for training, we incorporate prior knowledge into the generator input and supervision signals to make the adversarial model robust to small-scale training data.

Generator: Rather than using a Gaussian distributed vector as input like vanilla GANs, we carefully design a three-channel input for our generator as shown in Fig. 2. The first channel corresponds to a "normal" image that provides contextual information about the overall breast. The second channel consists of a lesion patch directly pasted into the "normal" image to provide the texture of the mass. The third channel is a binary mask indicating the location where we aim to blend the lesion, as a way to inform the model to pay more attention to this region. With these strong clues, we purposefully ease the task of our generative model, such that it can focus on the task of seamless blending alone. The generator is a fully convolutional network (FCN) that takes these three channels as input and produces an image with mass. The generator has an hourglass architecture with an encoder and a decoder. The encoder assimilates and fuses information associated with the normal breast and lesion patch. The decoder then expands the encoded information to generate a realistic image. In order to preserve the prior knowledge, we add the skip connections between the encoder and decoder layers to facilitate the propagation of prior clues given at the input.

Patch Discriminator: The generated images from the generator are then fed into a discriminator whose purpose is to verify the quality of the synthesized mammogram. In most existing GANs based method the discriminator performs an image level classification to distinguish real from fake images. However, in medical imaging, the texture details are crucial and a global classifier could overlook such information. We therefore propose to explore a patch discriminator [7] that can focus on the texture details in local image patches. This discriminator aims to classify whether each $N \times N$ patch in an image is real or fake. If a region looks fake or lacks texture details, it will result in a large value of loss forcing the generator to improve the quality. We run this discriminator convolutionally across the image and average all responses to provide the final output. In our experiments, we empirically set $N = 16$.

2.2   Adversarial Seamless Blending Supervision

Given a lesion patch E, a "normal" breast image X and a random position (x, y), the blending generator $\mathcal{G}$ aims to generate an artificial mammogram image $\tilde{Y}$ that contains the lesion at the position (x, y):

$$\tilde{Y} = \mathcal{G}(X, E, x, y; \theta_g)$$

where θ_g corresponds to the parameters of the network that should be optimized. Since our goal is to incorporate the lesion into a breast image, the network needs to pay attention to two parts: the region Ω where we want to integrate the lesion, and the remainder of the image, $\mathcal{B}$, where we want to keep unaltered (Fig. 3). The network needs to imagine how the lesion should grow according to the characteristics of the breast tissue inside the target region Ω, while keeping the background portion $\mathcal{B}$ identical. To this end, we propose the adversarial seamless blending supervision signals to guide the training process.

$$L = L_{adv} + \lambda_p L_{prior} \tag{1}$$

Adversarial Loss: We aim to generate synthetic images that are indistinguishable from real images, in order that the generated mammograms can be used as training samples. More specifically, we apply the adversarial loss [4] to supervise the generator and the discriminator in an adversarial manner:

$$L_{adv} = \mathbb{E}_Y[\log D(Y)] + \mathbb{E}_{X,E}[\log(1 - D(G(X,E)))] \qquad (2)$$

where the generator G is constrained to produce realistic images to confuse the discriminator D, while the discriminator D should correctly distinguish real images Y from generated ones $G(X,E)$. However, the min-max game between the generator and discriminator is not easy to converge during training, especially with a small-scale dataset. Therefore, we introduce the additional prior knowledge loss $L_{prior} = L_S + L_B$ to help guide the training process. It is composed of the following two loss functions and balanced with the parameter λ_p.

Seamless Blending Loss: As the lesions are often of small size in mammograms and the adversarial loss specifies only a high-level goal for the authenticity of the entire image, the generator may generate mammogram without any lesions. To circumvent this issue, we propose the following loss to make the generator pay attention to the region Ω where we aim to blend the lesion.

$$L_S = \|\nabla G(X,E)_\Omega - \mathbf{v}\|_2 \qquad (3)$$

where

$$\text{for all } i,j \in \Omega, \ \mathbf{v}(i,j) = \begin{cases} \nabla X_\Omega(i,j) & \text{if } |\nabla X_\Omega(i,j)| > |\nabla E(i,j)| \\ \nabla E(i,j) & \text{otherwise} \end{cases} \qquad (4)$$

This supervision signal makes the generator take into account the intensity variations of both the source lesion E and the normal tissue patch X_Ω for seamless blending. The notation $\nabla(\cdot)$ represents the gradient operation.

Background Loss: In order to preserve the background region $\mathcal{B}$ of the breast as given at input, we constrain the generator to output an image that maintains identical intensity and gradient. We employ both the L1 distance loss and the gradient difference loss to supervise the generator:

$$L_B = \|(G(X,E) - X)_\mathcal{B}\|_1 + \|(|\nabla G(X,E)| - |\nabla X|)_\mathcal{B}\|_2 \qquad (5)$$

The subscript $\mathcal{B}$ indicates that the supervision operates at the background region of the breast excluding the location where we aim to incorporate the lesion. We use L1 distance rather than L2 as the former encourages less blurring [7]. The gradient loss plays a complementary role to L1 loss and forces the generator to better preserve the texture variations in background regions.

Note that both the adversarial loss L_{adv} and the prior loss L_{prior} should be used together to ensure the quality of synthetic images. Without the adversarial loss, the generated images may lack the texture details and appear fake. Without the prior loss, the generator will not be able to perform the seamless blending.

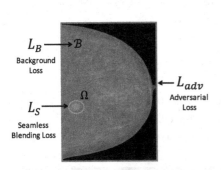

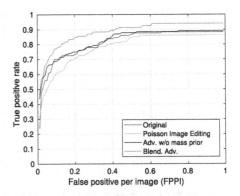

Fig. 3. Different regions on the image where the loss functions are applied. The background loss affects the background regions, the seamless blending loss focuses on the mass, and the adversarial loss controls the quality of the whole image.

Fig. 4. FROC curves comparing the detection performance of detectors trained with original data and complementary data generated by PIE, adv. w/o prior knowledge of mass and our blend. adv. methods, respectively.

2.3 Mass Localization

As training a detection model requires a large-amount of data, most existing deep learning based methods for breast cancer diagnosis using mammograms are limited to image-level classification [2,14,16]. In this paper, we adjust the state-of-the-art object detection framework, Mask R-CNN [5], for mass detection in mammography and improve the detection performance with our generated data. Note that recently more and more deep detector based methods have been proposed for mass detection, but they require large training datasets. Given an input mammogram, the proposed model aims to detect the lesion with both bounding boxes and segmentation masks. In addition to the classification loss and bounding box regression loss, we supervise the network with the segmentation loss to exploit pixel-wise information. The multi-task loss for each region of interest (RoI) is defined as:

$$L_{det} = L_{cls} + \lambda_{loc}L_{loc} + \lambda_{seg}L_{seg} \tag{6}$$

where L_{cls} is the classification loss, L_{loc} corresponds to the bounding box regression loss, and L_{seg} is the segmentation loss. λ_{loc} and λ_{seg} are weighting factors for different components of the loss function.

3   Experiments and Results

Database: We conducted our experiments on the widely used digital mammography dataset INbreaset [11]. This dataset comprises of a set of 115 cases containing 410 images, where 116 images contain benign or malignant masses.

Table 1. Comparison of detection performance with state-of-the-art methods in terms of true positive rate (TPR) versus false positive per image (FPPI) on INbreast dataset.

Method	TPR@FPPI	Run-time
Kozegar *et al.* [10]	0.65@1.1, 0.87@3.67	108 s
Dhungel *et al.* [1]	0.87 ± 0.14@0.8, 0.96 ± 0.03@1.2	20 s
Dhungel *et al.* [3]	0.90 ± 0.02@1.3, 0.95 ± 0.02@5.0	39 s
Jung *et al.* [8]	0.88 ± 0.07@0.5, 0.91 ± 0.07@1.3	1.8 s
Ours-Blend. Adv	0.91 ± 0.07@0.5, 0.94 ± 0.07@0.8	0.5 s

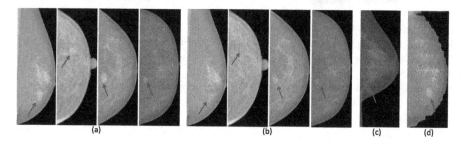

Fig. 5. Visualization of the images generated by (a) our blending adversarial networks, (b) Poisson image editing method, (c) adversarial model without mass prior knowledge and (d) vanilla GANs, respectively. The arrows indicate the position of the masses.

While INbreast is among the highest quality public mammography dataset with accurate annotations, there are only a limited number of images. We computed the results using a 5-fold cross validation experiment by carefully dividing the 115 cases into 80% for training and 20% for testing at the patient-level to avoid any positive bias.

Implementation Details: We adopted U-Net [13] as the backbone for our generator and a series of four convolutional layers for our patch discriminator. For our mass detector, we employed ResNet50 [6] as backbone and initialized the parameters with COCO pretrained model. To facilitate better convergence, the training process consists of three steps: (1) only the top layers are learned for the first 30 epochs, (2) all layers from stage 4 of ResNet are fine-tuned for 30 epochs, and (3) we optimize all layers for 40 epochs.

In order to test the ability of the model to localize lesions, we evaluate the predictions using the Free-Response Operating Characteristic curve (FROC). The FROC curve depicts the true positive rate as a function of the number of false positives per image (FPPI). A mass is considered to be correctly localized if the intersection over union (IoU) ratio between the ground truth bounding box and the predicted bounding box is higher than 0.5.

Results and Analysis: To evaluate how well the generated images can enhance the mass detector performance, we trained a few variants of the detector, using either the original data, or the original data plus one of three types of generated complementary data: (1) using conventional Poisson Image Editing (PIE) blending method [12]; (2) using an adversarial network without prior information of mass; and (3) using our blending adversarial networks. For each case, we generate 200 complementary data, making the training data approximately three times larger than original data set. For generating a mammogram with lesion, we randomly select a region in a "normal" breast mammogram and a real lesion as input for our generator. Note that we randomly resize and rotate the input lesion to augment the data.

The FROC curves in Fig. 4 depict the performance of the model trained with different sets of data. We can see that the detector trained with the additional data generated by our blending adversarial networks performs significantly better than the detector trained only with the original data. We observe an improvement of $\sim 10\%$ on the true positive rate for the same number of false positives per image, clearly demonstrating the effectiveness of the proposed method. Using the data generated by our blending adversarial networks as complementary training data makes the detector more robust due to expanded sample space of the training data. Some examples of the images generated by our blending adversarial networks are shown in Fig. 5(a).

On the other hand, we observe a degradation of performance when the detector is trained with the additional data generated by the conventional Poisson Image Editing method [12]. These results suggest that naively increasing the number of training images may potentially lead to adverse effects. The adversarial learning process guides our generator to approximate the underlying distribution of the authentic data. In contrast, the conventional image processing methods are unable to control the quality of the generated sample. As illustrated in Fig. 5(b), the lesions are often invisible in images synthesized with the PIE approach. This "over-blending" effect tends to mislead the detector. Furthermore, prior knowledge is crucial for learning a data generative model with a small-scale dataset. Figure 5(c) shows that without the prior knowledge of mass, *i.e.* replacing the real lesion patch with random noise at the input to the generator, the generated images lack fine texture details inside the mass region. Additionally, as shown in Fig. 5(d), the vanilla GANs (generating both breast and lesion from noise input) fail for dataset of this size and is only able to generate a mean shape of the breast with severe visual artifacts.

We compare the performance of our detector with several mass detection methods in the literature [1,8,10], and tabulate the results in Table 1. We follow the evaluation metrics as in previous works by giving the true positive rate at some acceptable false positive per image rates (TPR@FPPI). Our detector correctly localizes 91% of masses with a FPPI rate as of 0.50, while the existing mass detection approaches achieve similar true positive rates only with much larger number of false alarms. The run-time efficiency of the detector is also a key criterion for users. Without any cascaded structures or post refinement, our detector can execute at significantly higher speed of 0.5 s per image.

4   Conclusion

In this paper, we proposed blending adversarial networks to help address the issue of class imbalance and data scarcity in mammography. We made full use of the existing "normal" images to generate breast mammograms with synthetic masses that could be used as positive samples for training deep learning based mass detector. As testament to the effectiveness of the proposed method, extensive experiments on the widely-used INbreast dataset demonstrated significant improvement of the detection performance.

References

1. Dhungel, N., Carneiro, G., Bradley, A.P.: Automated mass detection in mammograms using cascaded deep learning and random forests. In: DICTA (2015)
2. Dhungel, N., Carneiro, G., Bradley, A.P.: The automated learning of deep features for breast mass classification from mammograms. In: Ourselin, S., Joskowicz, L., Sabuncu, M.R., Unal, G., Wells, W. (eds.) MICCAI 2016. LNCS, vol. 9901, pp. 106–114. Springer, Cham (2016). https://doi.org/10.1007/978-3-319-46723-8_13
3. Dhungel, N., Carneiro, G., Bradley, A.P.: A deep learning approach for the analysis of masses in mammograms with minimal user intervention. Med. Image Anal. **37**, 114–128 (2017)
4. Goodfellow, I., et al.: Generative adversarial nets. In: NIPS (2014)
5. He, K., Gkioxari, G., Dollár, P., Girshick, R.: Mask R-CNN. In: ICCV (2017)
6. He, K., Zhang, X., Ren, S., Sun, J.: Deep residual learning for image recognition. In: CVPR (2016)
7. Isola, P., Zhu, J.Y., Zhou, T., Efros, A.A.: Image-to-image translation with conditional adversarial networks. In: 2017 IEEE Conference on Computer Vision and Pattern Recognition (CVPR), pp. 5967–5976. IEEE (2017)
8. Jung, H., et al.: Detection of masses in mammograms using a one-stage object detector based on a deep convolutional neural network. PloS one **13**(9), e0203355 (2018)
9. Korkinof, D., Rijken, T., O'Neill, M., Yearsley, J., Harvey, H., Glocker, B.: High-resolution mammogram synthesis using progressive generative adversarial networks. arXiv preprint arXiv:1807.03401 (2018)
10. Kozegar, E., Soryani, M., Minaei, B., Domingues, I., et al.: Assessment of a novel mass detection algorithm in mammograms. J. Cancer Res. Ther. **9**(4), 592 (2013)
11. Moreira, I.C., Amaral, I., Domingues, I., Cardoso, A., Cardoso, M.J., Cardoso, J.S.: INbreast: toward a full-field digital mammographic database. Acad. Radiol. **19**(2), 236–248 (2012)
12. Pérez, P., Gangnet, M., Blake, A.: Poisson image editing. ACM TOG **22**(3), 313–318 (2003)
13. Ronneberger, O., Fischer, P., Brox, T.: U-Net: convolutional networks for biomedical image segmentation. In: Navab, N., Hornegger, J., Wells, W.M., Frangi, A.F. (eds.) MICCAI 2015. LNCS, vol. 9351, pp. 234–241. Springer, Cham (2015). https://doi.org/10.1007/978-3-319-24574-4_28

14. Shen, L.: End-to-end training for whole image breast cancer diagnosis using an all convolutional design. In: NIPS workshop (2017)
15. Wu, E., Wu, K., Cox, D., Lotter, W.: Conditional infilling GANs for data augmentation in mammogram classification. In: Stoyanov, D., et al. (eds.) RAMBO/BIA/TIA -2018. LNCS, vol. 11040, pp. 98–106. Springer, Cham (2018). https://doi.org/10.1007/978-3-030-00946-5_11
16. Zhu, W., Lou, Q., Vang, Y.S., Xie, X.: Deep multi-instance networks with sparse label assignment for whole mammogram classification. In: Descoteaux, M., Maier-Hein, L., Franz, A., Jannin, P., Collins, D.L., Duchesne, S. (eds.) MICCAI 2017. LNCS, vol. 10435, pp. 603–611. Springer, Cham (2017). https://doi.org/10.1007/978-3-319-66179-7_69

Tunable CT Lung Nodule Synthesis Conditioned on Background Image and Semantic Features

Ziyue Xu[✉], Xiaosong Wang, Hoo-Chang Shin, Holger Roth, Dong Yang,
Fausto Milletari, Ling Zhang, and Daguang Xu

Nvidia Corp., Bethesda, USA
ziyuex@nvidia.com

Abstract. Synthetic CT image with artificially generated lung nodules
has been shown to be useful as an augmentation method for certain tasks
such as lung segmentation and nodule classification. Most conventional
methods are designed as "inpainting" tasks by removing a region from
background image and synthesizing the foreground nodule. To ensure
natural blending with the background, existing method proposed loss
function and separate shape/appearance generation. However, spatial
discontinuity is still unavoidable for certain cases. Meanwhile, there is
often little control over semantic features regarding the nodule characteristics, which may limit their capability of fine-grained augmentation
in balancing the original data. In this work, we address these two challenges by developing a 3D multi-conditional generative adversarial network (GAN) that is conditioned on both background image and semantic
features for lung nodule synthesis on CT image. Instead of removing part
of the input image, we use a fusion block to blend object and background,
ensuring more realistic appearance. Multiple discriminator scenarios are
considered, and three outputs of image, segmentation, and feature are
used to guide the synthesis process towards semantic feature control. We
trained our method on public dataset, and showed promising results as
a solution for tunable lung nodule synthesis.

1 Introduction

Among the three major factors enabling the success of deep learning - data,
algorithm, and computation power, data covering sufficient population distribution is often most critical and most difficult to achieve. This is especially true
for medical image domain, in which labeled data availability is limited by its
unique characteristics: (1) medical images often involves high cost to produce,
and sensitivity in sharing; (2) pathological cases can have large variability in
appearances, and are often unbalanced/long tail in distribution; (3) accurate
labeling of the data requires high professional expertise, and can nevertheless
have large inter- and intra- observer variability even among experts.

Therefore, current work in medical domain mostly relies on using labeled
large public datasets [1], automated and/or semi-automated methods [5], and

© Springer Nature Switzerland AG 2019
N. Burgos et al. (Eds.): SASHIMI 2019, LNCS 11827, pp. 62–70, 2019.
https://doi.org/10.1007/978-3-030-32778-1_7

existing clinical report mining [12]. Recently, the development of generative adversarial networks (GAN) [2] has enabled a promising way in data augmentation: generate realistic synthetic data for training purpose. Preliminary works along this direction has demonstrated the potential of such approach in lung segmentation [6], brain tumor segmentation [11] and lung nodule classification [13].

Although shown to be promising, current GAN-based methods generate synthetic images based on limited information such as segmentation [8] and surrounding images [6]. Few recent works investigated finer control over the synthesis process, for example, controlling the malignancy property of the generated lung nodules [13]. However, to our best knowledge, there is no prior work that has the capability of controlling the semantic features of the synthesized nodules.

Meanwhile, most of previous methods model the synthesis process as an "inpainting" problem, in which a portion of the background image is removed before inpainting the synthesized nodule. One shortcoming of such model is that the fusion between synthetic region and background image may not be natural. To address this challenge, previous work used multi-mask reconstruction loss [6], or decoupled mask-appearance generation [8]. However, since the original information is lost in the background image input, it is difficult to recover the spatial continuity, even with the proposed methods.

In this work, we develop a 3D multi-conditional GAN model learning the shape and appearance distributions of lung nodules related to semantic features in 3D space. We aim to generate not only realistic but also tunable nodules according to its semantic features. Hence, our GAN is conditioned on both surrounding background information and a controllable feature set. In order to ensure a natural fusion with background image, we use two outputs of image and its corresponding nodule mask to reinforce the blending of the two, rather than erasing the region from base image. Multiple generator and discriminator losses are used to guide the network towards controlling the semantic feature inputs. We apply our strategy to public lung nodule dataset of LIDC [1], where each nodule is linked with a series of semantic annotations describing its appearances.

This work's main contributions are: (1) we synthesize 3D lung nodules and control its properties by using a 3D multi-conditional GAN with both surrounding images and semantic features; (2) instead of inpainting, we address the object/background fusion by multi-output and fusion block within network design; (3) both feature learning and fusion learning are performed by designing their corresponding outputs and losses during network training.

2   Method

To address the challenges of (1) incorporating semantic features, and (2) object/background fusion, inspired by works for 2D natural image synthesis [7,10], we design our network as a 3D multi-conditional GAN with style specification by additional regression branch. The generator takes in two conditions of background image and semantic feature, and produces three outputs of synthetic image, nodule mask, and predicted feature. The object/background fusion is performed with fusion blocks at each resolution level. The inter-relationships among background, semantic feature, and target nodule are controlled via multiple losses from generator and discriminator. Figures 1 and 2 depicts an overview of our method. Below, we outline the GAN architecture, loss function design, and training strategy for learning appearance together with the semantic features.

2.1   GAN Architecture

Figure 1 illustrates the structure of the proposed generator. Background image is encoded via a series of convolutional layers with three resolution levels, each downsampling doubles the feature channel. The semantic features are transformed via a fully connected layer and reshaped to bottleneck image size. The blending of object (nodule) and background image is performed via fusion block.

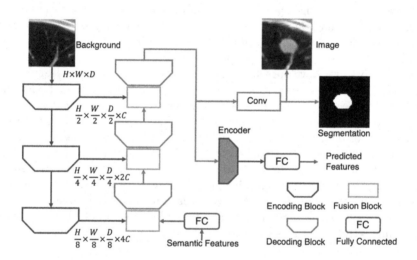

Fig. 1. Proposed generator of the 3D multi-conditional GAN for tunable nodule synthesis. Generator utilizes both background image and semantic feature code to synthesize image, nodule segmentation, and also a regression branch for feature code prediction.

As shown in Fig. 2, following [10], the fusion block is designed so that half of the object code is used to control the "soft" merging of the two feature sets in order to produce the synthetic image and its corresponding segmentation mask. Such fusion is enforced by the prediction of segmentation mask as an auxiliary output during training. As compared with "inpainiting", this strategy performs better in natural blending of the object/background. Also, the mask output is potentially helpful for data augmentation in tasks such as detection and segmentation.

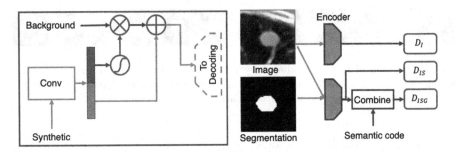

Fig. 2. Fusion block and discriminator of the 3D multi-conditional GAN. Left: fusion block at each resolution layer helps to fuse the information from background with that from previous layer. Right: with image, segmentation, and feature code, discriminator distinguishes three types of real/fake scenarios (Sect. 2.2).

To address the challenge of semantic feature specification, in addition to discriminator pairing, we added a regression branch (Fig. 1) beyond synthetic image and mask generation. Specifically, a encoding block is added to the output layer of the generator followed by fully connected layer to predict the vector of semantic features from the synthesized feature map. Furthermore, to control the size of the generated nodule, a loss is computed from the size of mask prediction in comparison with that of the ground truth segmentation of training data.

Figure 3 shows a result example for the proposed GAN from three views. The second column is the weighting mask from the last fusion block. It can be observed that the nodule and background are naturally separated and fused with the proposed fusion block and network.

2.2 Loss Functions and Training Strategy

The proposed GAN synthesize nodule with segmentation according to semantic feature vector. In order to guide the training process, several losses are proposed to supervise different aspects of the network.

The discriminator is illustrated in Fig. 2. The input to the discriminator is a tuple of image-segmentation-semantic feature code. Two encoders are utilized to encode: (1) image for discriminator D_I, and (2) image-segmentation pairs for discriminator D_{IS}. The second encoder's output is further combined with feature code f and further encoded via convolution, batch normalization, and leaky ReLU activation layers for discriminator D_{ISG}. Discriminators are trained with least squares loss functions [9]. Given image x, matched semantic feature code f, and matched segmentation mask m, tuples to be discriminated against it include cases containing mismatched feature code $\bar{f}$, mismatched segmentation mask $\bar{m}$, synthetic image G_x, and synthetic mask G_m. Let p_d and p_G denote the distributions of real and synthetic data, we have $x, f, m, \bar{f}, \bar{m} \sim p_d$ and

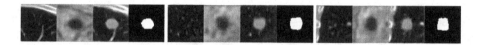

Fig. 3. Example of results produced by proposed synthesis GAN from three views: left to right - background image, background weight image during fusion, synthesized nodule image, and output segmentation mask.

$G_x, G_m \sim p_G$. With different combinations, we have

$$L_{D_I} = \mathbb{E}[(D_I(x) - 1)^2] + \mathbb{E}[D_I(G_x)^2]$$
$$L_{D_{IS}} = \mathbb{E}[(D_{IS}(x, m) - 1)^2] + \mathbb{E}[D_{IS}(x, \bar{m})^2] + \mathbb{E}[D_{IS}(G_x, G_m)^2]$$
$$L_{D_{ISG}} = \mathbb{E}[(D_{ISG}(x, m, f) - 1)^2] + \mathbb{E}[D_{ISG}(x, \bar{m}, f)^2]$$
$$+ \mathbb{E}[D_{ISG}(x, m, \bar{f})^2] + \mathbb{E}[D_{ISG}(G_x, G_m, f)^2]$$

For training the generator, in addition to discriminator loss, we further reinforced background reconstruction, semantic feature prediction, and size control with their corresponding losses. Let $G_{\bar{M}}$ be a morphological eroded version of segmentation mask G_m's inverse (i.e. background region), $\odot$ denote element-wise multiplication. The background reconstruction loss $L_{G_{BG}}$ is formulated as the $L1$ loss over background between synthetic image G_x and base image x. The semantic feature prediction loss L_{G_F} and size loss L_{G_s} are formulated as the $L2$ loss between predictions G_f, G_s and ground truth f, s, where $G_s = \sum(G_m > 0)$ and $s = \sum(m > 0)$

$$L_{G_{BG}} = \mathbb{E}[\|G_x \odot G_{\bar{M}} - x \odot G_{\bar{M}}\|_1]$$
$$L_{G_F} = \mathbb{E}[\|G_f - f\|_2]$$
$$L_{G_s} = \mathbb{E}[\|G_s - s\|_2]$$

With all the proposed losses, the generator loss is

$$L_G = \mathbb{E}[(D_I(G_x) - 1)^2] + \mathbb{E}[(D_{IS}(G_x, G_m) - 1)^2]$$
$$+ \mathbb{E}[(D_{ISG}(G_x, G_m, g) - 1)^2] + \lambda_1 L_{G_{BG}} + \lambda_2 L_{G_F} + \lambda_3 L_{G_S}$$

3 Experiment and Result

We evaluate the proposed method using the publicly available LIDC dataset [1]. This dataset contains 1018 chest CT scans of patients with lung nodules. There are 9 semantic features for each nodule: subtlety, internal structure, calcification, sphericity, margin, lobulation, spiculation, texture, and malignancy. Additionally, we can calculate the volume V of each nodule's manual segmentation, and estimate its diameter using sphere model $d = \sqrt[3]{6V/\pi}$. For this work, we select a subset of all nodules with approximate diameter between 3 mm and 30 mm following clinical standard of micro-nodule (<3 mm) and mass (>30 mm) [3]. In total there are 5942 semantic records from 826 patients. Note that multiple records can be related to the same nodule, as a single nodule can be annotated by several experts. Therefore, the annotation inherently contains certain amount of variability/noise. A $60 \times 60 \times 60$ mm^3 volume-of-interest (VOI) centered at each nodule is first cropped from the original image, then resampled to a fixed size of $64 \times 64 \times 64$.

To generate background image, we first: (1) segment the lung region of each CT volume using [4] from the whole CT volume; (2) make binary union of all manual nodule segmentations; and (3) exclude the nodule mask from lung mask. Hence there will be no nodule presence within the resulting mask after step (3), so that "painting nodule over existing nodule" can be avoided. Next, distance transform is computed from this mask, and centers for 3D background VOI patches are selected at a random location 5 to 25 mm from the mask boundary. The VOIs of the same size as nodule cases are cropped and resized to a fixed size of $64 \times 64 \times 64$.

The aim of our proposed method is to (1) generate realistic nodules and natural blending with the specified background, and (2) control the nodule appearance with semantic features.

Figure 4 shows the performance of image synthesis with multi-conditional GAN. As shown in the image, based on random nodule-free background B, the proposed method generates realistic images D, which reflects the semantic features as the reference training samples A (clear/fuzzy boundary, solid/ground-glass, etc.). As comparison, we implemented a 3D version of baseline [10], although it also have feature vector matching during discriminator phase, it failed to achieve same level of semantic feature control without the help of regression branch.

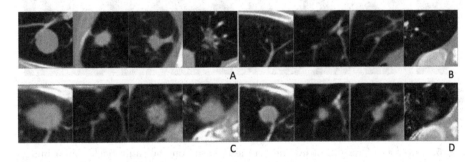

Fig. 4. Result of nodule synthesis, A: 4 different training image, B: random nodule-free background image, C: synthetic image generated by 3D version of baseline method [10], and D: synthetic images generated by the proposed method. Note that A, C, and D shared the same semantic features.

Figure 5 shows the synthesis result using the same background image with various semantic features and sizes. Two sets of examples are given under three views, and one additional result on changing size only is presented with one view (last row). As shown in the image, the proposed method has the capability of generating various nodules from a background image under different configurations of semantic features and sizes. From the result, we can observe some distortion of the background image, especially for the ground-glass, heterogeneous case of the last column due to its challenging nature. Last row shows the change with small to large size parameters. We observe that although the size changed as expected, they are not very accurate with regard to the real "expected" size (as input parameter). Therefore, potential improvements and future work include the investigation into annotation uncertainty/correlation among semantic features, better network structure design for higher quality image and more accurate control, and application to other tasks as data augmentation.

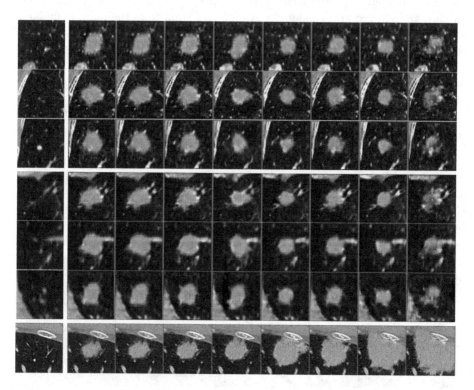

Fig. 5. Two sets of results of nodule synthesis based on the same background image under different semantic features and sizes, three views are provided. First column is the background image, and the following columns are synthetic cases, each column using a semantic feature/size combination. Last row showed an experiment of changing size parameter only.

4   Conclusion

We use a multi-conditional GAN, coupled with fusion structure, multiple outputs, and loss functions, to effectively generate realistic nodules with control over appearance by semantic features and size. Without erasing any portion of condition image, the proposed method achieves realistic nodule generation and smooth background fusion. The tunable size and semantic features ensures further diversified and targeted data augmentation. Current results showed promising diversity, however, more vigorous study is needed to verify their actual "controllability" over the image generation. As such, our approach can provide a potentially effective means for nodule image sample generation.

References

1. Armato III, S.G., McLennan, G., Bidaut, L., McNitt-Gray, M.F., Meyer, C.R., et al.: The lung image database consortium (LIDC) and image database resource initiative (IDRI): a completed reference database of lung nodules on CT scans. Med. Phys. **38**(2), 915–931 (2011)
2. Goodfellow, I., et al.: Generative adversarial nets. In: Advances in Neural Information Processing Systems, vol. 27, pp. 2672–2680 (2014)
3. Hansell, D.M., Bankier, A.A., MacMahon, H., McLoud, T.C., Mller, N.L., Remy, J.: Fleischner society: glossary of terms for thoracic imaging. Radiology **246**(3), 697–722 (2008)
4. Harrison, A.P., Xu, Z., George, K., Lu, L., Summers, R.M., Mollura, D.J.: Progressive and multi-path holistically nested neural networks for pathological lung segmentation from CT images. In: Descoteaux, M., Maier-Hein, L., Franz, A., Jannin, P., Collins, D.L., Duchesne, S. (eds.) MICCAI 2017. LNCS, vol. 10435, pp. 621–629. Springer, Cham (2017). https://doi.org/10.1007/978-3-319-66179-7_71
5. Jin, D., Xu, Z., Harrison, A.P., George, K., Mollura, D.J.: 3D convolutional neural networks with graph refinement for airway segmentation using incomplete data labels. In: Wang, Q., Shi, Y., Suk, H.-I., Suzuki, K. (eds.) MLMI 2017. LNCS, vol. 10541, pp. 141–149. Springer, Cham (2017). https://doi.org/10.1007/978-3-319-67389-9_17
6. Jin, D., Xu, Z., Tang, Y., Harrison, A.P., Mollura, D.J.: CT-realistic lung nodule simulation from 3D conditional generative adversarial networks for robust lung segmentation. In: Frangi, A.F., Schnabel, J.A., Davatzikos, C., Alberola-López, C., Fichtinger, G. (eds.) MICCAI 2018. LNCS, vol. 11071, pp. 732–740. Springer, Cham (2018). https://doi.org/10.1007/978-3-030-00934-2_81
7. Karras, T., Laine, S., Aila, T.: A style-based generator architecture for generative adversarial networks. CoRR abs/1812.04948 (2018)
8. Liu, S., et al.: Decompose to manipulate: manipulable object synthesis in 3D medical images with structured image decomposition. CoRR abs/1812.01737 (2018)
9. Mao, X., Li, Q., Xie, H., Lau, R.Y.K., Wang, Z., Smolley, S.P.: Least squares generative adversarial networks. In: 2017 IEEE International Conference on Computer Vision (ICCV), pp. 2813–2821, October 2017
10. Park, H., Yoo, Y., Kwak, N.: MC-GAN: multi-conditional generative adversarial network for image synthesis. In: The British MachineVision Conference (BMVC) (2018)

11. Shin, H.-C., et al.: Medical image synthesis for data augmentation and anonymization using generative adversarial networks. In: Gooya, A., Goksel, O., Oguz, I., Burgos, N. (eds.) SASHIMI 2018. LNCS, vol. 11037, pp. 1–11. Springer, Cham (2018). https://doi.org/10.1007/978-3-030-00536-8_1
12. Wang, X., Peng, Y., Lu, L., Lu, Z., Bagheri, M., Summers, R.M.: ChestX-ray8: hospital-scale chest X-ray database and benchmarks on weakly-supervised classification and localization of common thorax diseases. In: The IEEE Conference on Computer Vision and Pattern Recognition (CVPR), July 2017
13. Yang, J., et al.: Class-aware adversarial lung nodule synthesis in CT images. CoRR abs/1812.11204 (2018)

Mask2Lesion: Mask-Constrained Adversarial Skin Lesion Image Synthesis

Kumar Abhishek$^{(\boxtimes)}$ and Ghassan Hamarneh

School of Computing Science, Simon Fraser University, Burnaby, Canada
{kabhishe,hamarneh}@sfu.ca

Abstract. Skin lesion segmentation is a vital task in skin cancer diagnosis and further treatment. Although deep learning based approaches have significantly improved the segmentation accuracy, these algorithms are still reliant on having a large enough dataset in order to achieve adequate results. Inspired by the immense success of generative adversarial networks (GANs), we propose a GAN-based augmentation of the original dataset in order to improve the segmentation performance. In particular, we use the segmentation masks available in the training dataset to train the Mask2Lesion model, and use the model to generate new lesion images given any arbitrary mask, which are then used to augment the original training dataset. We test Mask2Lesion augmentation on the ISBI ISIC 2017 Skin Lesion Segmentation Challenge dataset and achieve an improvement of 5.17% in the mean Dice score as compared to a model trained with only classical data augmentation techniques.

Keywords: Skin lesion · Generative adversarial networks · Image segmentation

1 Introduction

Melanoma, a type of skin cancer, although represents a small fraction of all skin cancers in the USA, accounts for over 75% of all skin cancer related fatalities [21], and is responsible for over 10,000 deaths annually across the country [1]. However, studies have shown that the survival rates of patients improve drastically with early diagnosis. Efficient assessment of dermoscopic images for indicators of melanoma is an important component of early diagnosis and improved patient prognosis. Automated methods to extract image features indicative of skin lesions are promising tools for dermatologists. Based on core methods such as the 7-point checklist [15], the ABCD (Asymmetry, Border, Color, and Differential structure) rule [18], and the CASH (Color, Architecture, Symmetry, and Homogeneity) algorithm [11], deep learning methods can aid the diagnosis of skin lesion images. However, these methods use hand-crafted features, and therefore rely on an accurate segmentation of the lesion [2]. Moreover, lesion segmentations have been used to assist melanoma diagnosis [12,23,26]. This motivates

© Springer Nature Switzerland AG 2019
N. Burgos et al. (Eds.): SASHIMI 2019, LNCS 11827, pp. 71–80, 2019.
https://doi.org/10.1007/978-3-030-32778-1_8

the use of deep learning based computer-aided diagnosis systems to improve the accuracy and sensitivity of melanoma detection methods.

Recent works on skin lesion segmentation using deep learning have shown significant improvements in segmentation accuracy. Yuan et al. [28] used a 19-layer deep fully convolutional network with a Jaccard distance based loss function that is trained end-to-end to segment skin lesions. Mirikharaji et al. [17] proposed a deep auto-context architecture to use image appearance information along with the contextual information to improve segmentation results. Yu et al. [27] proposed using a deep residual network architecture with several blocks stacked together to improve the representative capability of the network and therefore increased the segmentation accuracy.

Generative adversarial networks (GANs), proposed by Goodfellow et al. [9] have been immensely popular in realistic image generation tasks. Numerous variations of these generative models have been developed for a variety of applications, including text to image synthesis and video generation [20,24]. GANs have also been used to generate medical images of various modalities, such as generating liver lesion images to augment the CT lesion classification training dataset [8], generating chest X-ray images to augment the dataset for abnormality detection [16], and generating brain CT images from corresponding brain MR images [25]. Some skin lesion synthesis tasks have also relied upon GAN-based approaches, such as generating images of benign and malignant skin lesions [3], modeling skin lesions using semantic label maps and superpixels in order to generate new lesion images [6], and generating skin lesions along with their corresponding segmentation masks [19].

In this work, we propose to use lesion masks to generate synthetic lesion images in order to augment the segmentation training dataset and improve skin lesion segmentation performance. Isola et al. [13] and Zhu et al. [30] have shown that it is possible to generate high resolution realistic images from object boundaries. An inherent advantage of using lesion masks to generate skin lesion images is that the newly generated images can be used for training the segmentation network without requiring annotation. To the best of our knowledge, this is the first work towards generating skin lesion images from lesion masks.

The paper is structured as follows: we discuss the proposed approach in Sect. 2, describe the dataset and experimental details in Sect. 3, and analyze the quantitative and qualitative results of our proposed approach in Sect. 4. Section 5 concludes the paper.

2   Method

2.1   Method Overview

The purpose of our method is to synthesize segmentation training data which is then used to augment the existing data for training a segmentation network. We model this as an image-to-image translation task where we train a deep neural network model, called Mask2Lesion, to generate the synthetic data. In particular, we translate images containing binary segmentation masks, which highlight the area of a target skin lesion, to a skin image containing a lesion confined to that binary mask, making it a paired image-to-image translation task. To this end, we train a network with skin lesion images and their corresponding masks. Such training data is also typically provided for training segmentation methods. Our deep network is based on the pix2pix conditional generative adversarial network (GAN), described in Sect. 2.3. With the ability to translate a binary mask to a corresponding image containing a lesion delineated by the mask, we can then turn our attention to creating synthesized masks (via different approaches), and rely on our trained Mask2Lesion model to generate the corresponding images. Given a training dataset of images and segmentation masks, with or without augmentation (performed using Mask2Lesion or otherwise), we can then train a segmentation network. The segmentation network used here is described in Sect. 3.

2.2   Segmentation Masks

We propose to use lesion segmentation masks as input to the generative algorithm, making it easy to produce a large number of inputs. Since the ISIC 2017 Skin Lesion Segmentation Challenge dataset [7] used for the segmentation task has ground truth segmentation masks available, they can be used as inputs to the generative algorithm to synthesize skin lesions, thus creating new pairs of lesion images and their masks. Figure 1 shows four sample lesion images with their corresponding segmentation masks.

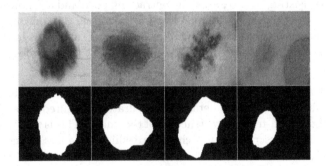

Fig. 1. A few sample images from the ISIC training dataset along with the corresponding segmentation masks. Note the presence of artifacts in some of the images.

2.3   Image-to-Image Translation Network

The paired image-to-image translation model proposed by Isola et al. [13] uses a conditional GAN to generate images. Unlike traditional GANs which learn a mapping from a random noise vector to an output image, conditional GANs learn a mapping from an observed image x and a random noise vector z to an output image y. The two components of a conditional GAN are a generator and a discriminator. The generator G is trained to produce output images, $G : \{x, z\} \to y$ which are "realistic", meaning they cannot be distinguished from the original images. The discriminator D tries to distinguish between the original images and the output of the generator G. The two components can be estimated using deep neural networks. This conditional GAN is trained in an adversarial manner, and the objective function can be written as

$$\mathcal{L}_{cGAN}(G, D) = \mathbb{E}_{x,y} \left[\log D(x, y)\right] + \mathbb{E}_{x,z} \left[\log \left(1 - D(x, G(x, z))\right)\right], \quad (1)$$

where the generator G tries to minimize this objective function and the discriminator D tries to maximize it. The optimal solution is obtained using this minimax game

$$G^* = \arg\min_{G} \ \arg\max_{D} \ \mathcal{L}_{cGAN}(G, D). \quad (2)$$

This is different from an unconditional GAN where the discriminator D does not observe the input image x.

Generator Architecture: Since the output of the generator shares the underlying structure with the input, an encoder decoder architecture with skip connections has been chosen as the generator. We use U-Net [22] with an L1 loss because, in its attempt to fool the discriminator, L2 loss tends to produce more blurry generator outputs. The U-Net has a fully convolutional neural network architecture consisting of two paths - a contracting path and a symmetric expansive path. Skip-connections containing feature maps from the contracting path to the symmetrically corresponding layer's upsampled feature maps in the expanding path assist recovery of the full spatial resolution at the network output [14].

Discriminator Architecture: While using the L1 loss for the generator ensures that the low frequency details are accurately captured, it is also important to model the high-frequency structure of the image. This is achieved by using a PatchGAN [13], a discriminator architecture which penalizes structure at local image patch level. As a result, the image is divided into several (overlapping) patches, each of which is labeled by the discriminator as "real" or "fake", and the overall output of the discriminator is the average of the individual responses. Fig. 2 shows a high level overview of the Mask2Lesion algorithm.

3   Data and Experimental Details

The dataset used for evaluation of the proposed approach was obtained from the 2017 ISBI ISIC Skin Lesion Analysis Towards Melanoma Detection: Lesion Segmentation Challenge [7], and contains 2000 training images and 150 test images. All the images and their corresponding ground truth segmentation masks

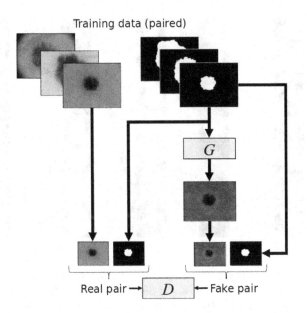

Fig. 2. The proposed Mask2Lesion algorithm.

were resized to 128×128 pixels using nearest neighbor interpolation from the SciPy library.

The Mask2Lesion model was trained for 200 epochs. For both the generator and the discriminator, all convolution operations used 4×4 spatial filters with a stride of 2. Each convolution layer (except the first) consists of convolution, batch normalization, dropout (with a keep probability of 0.5), and ReLU activation. The encoder (the contracting path of the U-Net) uses leaky ReLUs with a slope of 0.2, while the decoder (the expansive path) uses ReLUs. For the PatchGAN, a 70×70 patch is processed from the input image, which assigns a score to a 30×30 patch of the image.

As the goal of this work is to demonstrate the efficacy of the proposed Mask2Lesion model in augmenting the dataset for segmentation, we use U-Net [22] as a baseline segmentation network, and optimize it with mini-batch stochastic gradient descent with a batch size of 32. In order to evaluate the segmentation performance with and without GAN based augmentation, we train and evaluate four segmentation networks, and we use the following abbreviations to denote them while reporting results: (i) **NoAug:** trained on only the original training dataset without any augmentation, (ii) **ClassicAug:** trained on the original training dataset augmented with classical augmentation techniques (rotation, flipping, etc.), (iii) **Mask2LesionAug:** trained on the original training dataset augmented with Mask2Lesion outputs on masks from the training dataset, and (iv) **AllAug:** trained on the original dataset augmented with classical augmentation as well as Mask2Lesion outputs on masks from the training

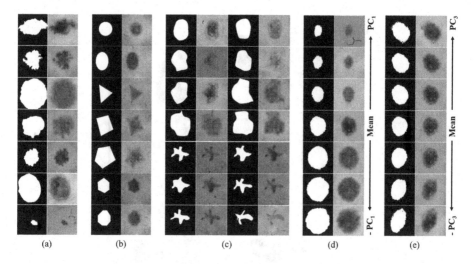

Fig. 3. (a) Segmentation masks from the ISIC dataset fed to Mask2Lesion and the corresponding generated lesion images. (b) Simple geometric shapes as masks and the corresponding outputs. (c) Elastic deformations applied to hand drawn masks using DeformIt and the corresponding synthesized lesion images. (d), (e) PCA-based deformations applied to segmentation masks and the corresponding Mask2Lesion outputs.

dataset. For all the segmentation networks, we report the metrics used in the challenge [7] - Dice coefficient, sensitivity, specificity, and pixel-wise accuracy.

4   Results and Discussion

We use the segmentation masks from the ISIC dataset as inputs to the Mask2Lesion model, and the corresponding generated lesion images are shown in Fig. 3(a). We see that the synthesized lesions express variance in appearances and textures.

Next, we test Mask2Lesion by using simple geometric shapes as masks, showing that synthesized images are well constrained by the mask boundaries (Fig. 3(b)). We also test the adaptability of Mask2Lesion to hand-drawn masks. We draw two shapes - a large blob and a star shape, and then apply varying degrees of elastic deformations to them using DeformIt [10]. These masks are then used as inputs to the Mask2Lesion model and the corresponding outputs are shown in Fig. 3(c). Furthermore, we apply deformations using a PCA-based shape model to segmentation masks. In particular, we generate new masks by weighting the first and the third principal components in the range $[-1, 1]$ in order to incorporate size and orientation changes (Fig. 3(d) and (e) respectively), and use these to generate lesion images. We note that the goal for testing on geometric shapes, hand-drawn masks, and masks deformed using PCA-based shape modeling is to showcase our method's ability to generate skin lesion images confined to the user-specified input masks, regardless of their complexity.

Table 1 shows the quantitative results for the test images evaluated using the four trained segmentation networks. We see that Mask2LesionAug outperforms ClassicAug in Dice coefficient, sensitivity, and specificity. Moreover, AllAug (which combines both classical as well as Mask2Lesion-based augmentation) outperforms ClassicAug in all four metrics, and achieves a 5.17% improvement in the mean Dice coefficient. Figure 4 shows samples from the test dataset for which the segmentation accuracy significantly improved with AllAug. The outputs of AllAug are much more closer to the respective ground truths and have fewer false positives as compared to ClassicAug. Moreover, the segmentation performance is within a small margin of the top 3 entries on the challenge leaderboard [4, 5, 29] without using any pre-processing, post-processing or an ensemble of models [4, 29] or additional external data [5].

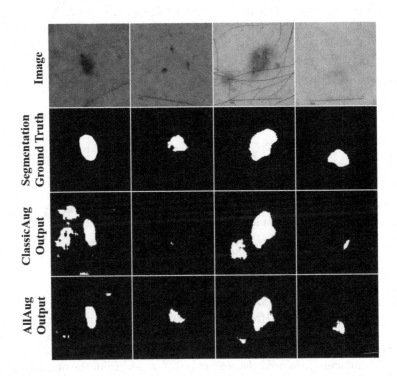

Fig. 4. Improved segmentation accuracy with AllAug. The first row shows the test image samples, the second row shows the segmentation ground truths and the third and the fourth rows show the segmentations obtained from the ClassicAug and AllAug respectively.

To further capture the segmentation performance improvement, we plot the Gaussian kernel density estimates of the Dice coefficient, the sensitivity, and the specificity obtained for the test images for the ClassicAug and AllAug (Fig. 5). The plots have been clipped to the range of values of the respective metrics and represent their probability density function estimates. The plots show higher peaks (which correspond to higher densities) at larger values of all the three

Table 1. Quantitative results for segmentation (Mean ± standard error)

Method		NoAug	ClassicAug	Mask2LesionAug	AllAug
Aug.	Classical	✗	✓	✗	✓
Method	Mask2Lesion	✗	✗	✓	✓
Dice		0.7723 ± 0.0185	0.7743 ± 0.0203	0.7849 ± 0.0160	**0.8144 ± 0.0160**
Accuracy		0.9316 ± 0.0089	0.9321 ± 0.0086	0.9311 ± 0.0087	**0.9375 ± 0.0091**
Sensitivity		0.7798 ± 0.0211	0.8094 ± 0.0222	0.8197 ± 0.0186	**0.8197 ± 0.0182**
Specificity		0.9744 ± 0.0035	0.9672 ± 0.0047	0.9698 ± 0.0045	**0.9762 ± 0.0038**

metrics for AllAug as compared to ClassicAug. Moreover, the range of the specificity of AllAug is smaller than that of ClassicAug, meaning that combining classical augmentation with Mask2Lesion-based augmentation results in fewer mislabeled pixels.

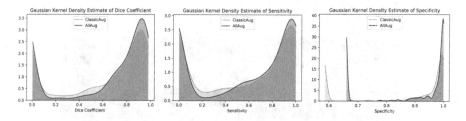

Fig. 5. Evaluating the proposed method - comparing Dice coefficient (left), sensitivity (middle), and specificity (right) for ClassicAug and AllAug.

5   Conclusion

In this work, we proposed Mask2Lesion, a conditional GAN-based model to generate skin lesion images from and constrained to binary masks, and used these newly generated images along with their corresponding masks to augment the training dataset for improving the segmentation accuracy of skin lesion images. In particular, we used the segmentation masks from the original dataset as input to the generative algorithm so as to avoid the manual annotation of the newly synthesized skin lesion images. We demonstrated that the generated lesion images are well-confined within the input mask boundaries, irrespective of the complexity of the masks. Our results showed a significant improvement in the segmentation accuracy when the training dataset for the segmentation network is augmented with these generated images. Future work directions include extending this model to generate skin lesion images with dermoscopic features as well as generating diagnosis label specific skin lesions.

Acknowledgements. Partial funding for this project is provided by the Natural Sciences and Engineering Research Council of Canada (NSERC). The authors are grateful to the NVIDIA Corporation for donating Titan X GPUs used in this research.

References

1. Cancer Facts & Figures (2016). https://www.cancer.org/research/cancer-facts-statistics/all-cancer-facts-figures/cancer-facts-figures-2016.html
2. Barata, C., Celebi, M.E., Marques, J.S.: A survey of feature extraction in dermoscopy image analysis of skin cancer. IEEE JBHI **23**(3), 1096–1109 (2018)
3. Baur, C., Albarqouni, S., Navab, N.: Generating highly realistic images of skin lesions with GANs. In: Stoyanov, D., et al. (eds.) CARE/CLIP/OR 2.0/ISIC - 2018. LNCS, vol. 11041, pp. 260–267. Springer, Cham (2018). https://doi.org/10.1007/978-3-030-01201-4_28
4. Berseth, M.: ISIC 2017-skin lesion analysis towards melanoma detection. arXiv preprint arXiv:1703.00523 (2017)
5. Bi, L., Kim, J., Ahn, E., Feng, D.: Automatic skin lesion analysis using large-scale dermoscopy images and deep residual networks. arXiv preprint arXiv:1703.04197 (2017)
6. Bissoto, A., Perez, F., Valle, E., Avila, S.: Skin lesion synthesis with generative adversarial networks. In: Stoyanov, D., et al. (eds.) CARE/CLIP/OR 2.0/ISIC - 2018. LNCS, vol. 11041, pp. 294–302. Springer, Cham (2018). https://doi.org/10.1007/978-3-030-01201-4_32
7. Codella, N.C., et al.: Skin lesion analysis toward melanoma detection: a challenge at the 2017 international symposium on biomedical imaging (ISBI), hosted by the international skin imaging collaboration (ISIC). In: ISBI, pp. 168–172 (2018)
8. Frid-Adar, M., Klang, E., Amitai, M., Goldberger, J., Greenspan, H.: Synthetic data augmentation using GAN for improved liver lesion classification. In: ISBI, pp. 289–293, April 2018
9. Goodfellow, I., et al.: Generative adversarial nets. In: NeurIPS, pp. 2672–2680 (2014)
10. Hamarneh, G., Jassi, P., Tang, L.: Simulation of ground-truth validation data via physically- and statistically-based warps. In: Metaxas, D., Axel, L., Fichtinger, G., Székely, G. (eds.) MICCAI 2008. LNCS, vol. 5241, pp. 459–467. Springer, Heidelberg (2008). https://doi.org/10.1007/978-3-540-85988-8_55
11. Henning, J.S., et al.: The CASH (color, architecture, symmetry, and homogeneity) algorithm for dermoscopy. J. Am. Acad. Dermatol. **56**(1), 45–52 (2007)
12. Hosny, K.M., Kassem, M.A., Foaud, M.M.: Classification of skin lesions using transfer learning and augmentation with Alex-net. PLoS One **14**(5), e0217293 (2019)
13. Isola, P., Zhu, J., Zhou, T., Efros, A.A.: Image-to-image translation with conditional adversarial networks. In: CVPR, pp. 5967–5976, July 2017
14. Li, H., Xu, Z., Taylor, G., Studer, C., Goldstein, T.: Visualizing the loss landscape of neural nets. In: NeurIPS, pp. 6389–6399 (2018)
15. Mackie, R., Doherty, V.: Seven-point checklist for melanoma. Clin. Exp. Dermatol. **16**(2), 151–152 (1991)
16. Madani, A., Moradi, M., Karargyris, A., Syeda-Mahmood, T.: Chest x-ray generation and data augmentation for cardiovascular abnormality classification. In: Medical Imaging 2018: Image Processing, vol. 10574, p. 105741M. International Society for Optics and Photonics (2018)
17. Mirikharaji, Z., Izadi, S., Kawahara, J., Hamarneh, G.: Deep auto-context fully convolutional neural network for skin lesion segmentation. In: ISBI, pp. 877–880 (2018)
18. Nachbar, F., et al.: The ABCD rule of dermatoscopy: high prospective value in the diagnosis of doubtful melanocytic skin lesions. J. Am. Acad. Dermatol. **30**(4), 551–559 (1994)

19. Pollastri, F., Bolelli, F., Paredes, R., Grana, C.: Augmenting data with GANs to segment melanoma skin lesions. Multimed. Tools Appl. 1–18 (2019). https://doi.org/10.1007/s11042-019-7717-y

20. Reed, S.E., Akata, Z., Yan, X., Logeswaran, L., Schiele, B., Lee, H.: Generative adversarial text to image synthesis. CoRR abs/1605.05396 (2016)

21. Rogers, H.W., Weinstock, M.A., Feldman, S.R., Coldiron, B.M.: Incidence estimate of nonmelanoma skin cancer (keratinocyte carcinomas) in the US population, 2012. JAMA Dermatol. **151**(10), 1081–1086 (2015)

22. Ronneberger, O., Fischer, P., Brox, T.: U-net: convolutional networks for biomedical image segmentation. In: Navab, N., Hornegger, J., Wells, W.M., Frangi, A.F. (eds.) MICCAI 2015. LNCS, vol. 9351, pp. 234–241. Springer, Cham (2015). https://doi.org/10.1007/978-3-319-24574-4_28

23. Sumithra, R., Suhil, M., Guru, D.: Segmentation and classification of skin lesions for disease diagnosis. Proc. Comput. Sci. **45**, 76–85 (2015)

24. Vondrick, C., Pirsiavash, H., Torralba, A.: Generating videos with scene dynamics. CoRR abs/1609.02612 (2016)

25. Wolterink, J.M., Dinkla, A.M., Savenije, M.H.F., Seevinck, P.R., van den Berg, C.A.T., Išgum, I.: Deep MR to CT synthesis using unpaired data. In: Tsaftaris, S.A., Gooya, A., Frangi, A.F., Prince, J.L. (eds.) SASHIMI 2017. LNCS, vol. 10557, pp. 14–23. Springer, Cham (2017). https://doi.org/10.1007/978-3-319-68127-6_2

26. Yan, Y., Kawahara, J., Hamarneh, G.: Melanoma recognition via visual attention. In: IPMI, pp. 793–804 (2019)

27. Yu, L., Chen, H., Dou, Q., Qin, J., Heng, P.A.: Automated melanoma recognition in dermoscopy images via very deep residual networks. IEEE TMI **36**(4), 994–1004 (2017)

28. Yuan, Y., Chao, M., Lo, Y.: Automatic skin lesion segmentation using deep fully convolutional networks with Jaccard distance. IEEE TMI **36**(9), 1876–1886 (2017)

29. Yuan, Y.: Automatic skin lesion segmentation with fully convolutional-deconvolutional networks. arXiv preprint arXiv:1703.05165 (2017)

30. Zhu, J.Y., Park, T., Isola, P., Efros, A.A.: Unpaired image-to-image translation using cycle-consistent adversarial networks. In: ICCV, pp. 2223–2232 (2017)

Towards Annotation-Free Segmentation of Fluorescently Labeled Cell Membranes in Confocal Microscopy Images

Dennis Eschweiler$^{(\boxtimes)}$, Tim Klose, Florian Nicolas Müller-Fouarge,
Marcin Kopaczka, and Johannes Stegmaier$^{(\boxtimes)}$

Institute of Imaging and Computer Vision, RWTH Aachen University,
Aachen, Germany
{dennis.eschweiler,johannes.stegmaier}@lfb.rwth-aachen.de

Abstract. The lack of labeled training data is one of the major challenges in the era of big data and deep learning. Especially for large and complex images, the acquisition of expert annotations becomes infeasible and although many microscopy images contain repetitive and regular structures, manual annotation effort remains expensive. To this end, we propose an approach to obtain image slices and corresponding annotations for confocal microscopy images showing fluorescently labeled cell membranes in an automated and unsupervised manner. Due to their regular structure, cell membrane positions are modeled in silico and respective raw images are synthesized by generative deep learning approaches. The resulting synthesized data set is validated based on the authenticity of generated images and the utilizability for training an existing deep learning segmentation approach. We show, that segmentation accuracy nearly reaches state-of-the-art performance for fluorescently labeled cell membranes in *A.thaliana*, without the expense of manual labeling.

Keywords: Cell membranes · Synthesis · Microscopy · Annotation-free

1 Introduction

In developmental biology, a large variety of cellular characteristics can be studied by analysis of cell shapes. Obtaining precise manual segmentations of cell membranes for detailed morphological analysis are a tedious task, due to large image sizes, proximity of cells and vanishing fluorescence intensities in deeper tissue layers. Poor or missing manual annotations limit the performance of learning-based segmentation approaches, especially in challenging image regions [3,6], which could be partly improved by the incorporation of deep learning methods [2,9]. However, in order to leverage the power of recent deep learning approaches and to train generalized models, large amounts of data are required. Reducing

---

D. Eschweiler and T. Klose—Authors contributed equally to this work.

© Springer Nature Switzerland AG 2019
N. Burgos et al. (Eds.): SASHIMI 2019, LNCS 11827, pp. 81–89, 2019.
https://doi.org/10.1007/978-3-030-32778-1_9

labeling expense and still obtaining enough annotations, is often accomplished by data augmentation [5] or sparse annotations [13]. Since augmentations have to remain in biological appropriate ranges, the amount and variety of data is limited and often can not account for generalized models. Transfer learning approaches overcome this issue by training models on large data sets from slightly related domains and only use small portions of labeled data from the target domain to fine-tune the model [5].

Both approaches, however, can not completely diminish the need for manual annotations. To achieve complete independence from manual interaction, data needs to be synthesized, which has been addressed for several biological experiments. Those approaches range from physical modeling of cells to generation of images based on classical image features [8,10,11]. More recently, generative adversarial approaches proved to achieve good results for data augmentations [5], as well as data generation [4,7].

Although previous methods work well for cell synthesis, they can not straightforwardly be adapted to work for cell membranes, which comprise a fundamentally different appearance. We propose a method, which approximates the complex, densely connected membrane network, by combining randomly sampled points and Voronoi diagrams. Subsequently, generative deep learning models are used to translate the obtained membrane segmentation to the image domain.

The main contributions of this work are (1) a parametrized generation of membrane segmentations and (2) unsupervised translation of the generated annotations to the image domain, by (3) using structure-aware losses, which ensure matching membrane locations in the label and image domain. Furthermore, (4) the proposed method offers a way to generate complete segmentations, even in regions of low or vanishing fluorescence signals, which constitute the most challenging and time-consuming regions for manual annotators.

For validation, we used annotated 2D slices (Fig. 1) of microscopy images showing fluorescently labeled cell membranes in *Arabidopsis thaliana* [12] and generated three additional data sets with different levels of abstraction. For each data set, authenticity of generated images, as well as utilizability for training of an existing segmentation approach [2] were assessed.

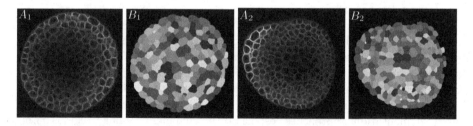

Fig. 1. (*A*) Cropped 2D slices from a 3D confocal image stack of fluorescently labeled cell membranes in *A. thaliana* and (*B*) the associated multi-instance segmentation [12].

2   Method

The proposed method follows a top-down approach by generating annotations first and subsequently synthesizing corresponding images. In this manner, the availability of complete annotations can be ensured and we are able to obtain images with arbitrary fluorescence intensity without losing information about true labels, even in regions of vanishing fluorescence signals. The proposed method can be divided into two sub-tasks, namely automated label generation and translation of labels to the image domain.

2.1   Label Generation

As shown in [2], generation of final instance segmentations can be improved by introducing an intermediate step that reformulates the instance segmentation problem as a 3-class semantic segmentation, dividing the image into background, membrane positions and cell centroids. This alternative representation describes annotations in a more general way and is utilized as baseline for synthesized annotations. As initial step, an arbitrary but plausible specimen shape is generated, dividing the image into foreground and background. Within the foreground region, rough cell locations are modeled by a predefined number of points n_{points} at randomly sampled positions. To prevent points from being too close to one another and generating unnatural changes of size among neighbouring cells, a k-means clustering approach is utilized. Clustering is performed for a predefined number of iterations n_{iter}, which allows to further control uniformity of distances between cell centroids. Based on these resulting cell positions, a Voronoi diagram is constructed to partition the foreground region into separated instances, with each of them representing a single cell. Therefore, morphological cell appearance and final cell count is parametrized by the parameter tuple $(n_{points}, n_{iter}, k)$.

2.2   Image Synthesis

To transfer the generated labels into a realistic-looking image domain, a cyclic generative adversarial network (cycleGAN) is utilized, which allows to perform domain transfers without the need of paired examples [14]. The underlying framework contains two generator networks and two discriminator networks, which are trained in an adversarial way. Considering data from the label domain $x_L \in \mathcal{X}_L$ and data from the image domain $x_I \in \mathcal{X}_I$, the generators contribute two mappings $G_{LI} : \mathcal{X}_L \mapsto \mathcal{X}_I$ and $G_{IL} : \mathcal{X}_I \mapsto \mathcal{X}_L$. The discriminator D_L aims to discriminate between reference samples x_L and translated samples $G_{IL}(x_I)$, whereas discriminator D_I discriminates between reference samples x_I and translated samples $G_{LI}(x_L)$.

Network architectures for generators and discriminators are adapted from [14] and comprise a residual-based architecture for generators, which operate on input patches of size 256×256 pixel and PatchGANs are used as discriminators.

As introduced in [14], the framework is trained by optimizing different loss terms, namely the adversarial loss $\mathcal{L}_{GAN}$, the cycle-consistency loss $\mathcal{L}_{cyc}$ and the identity loss $\mathcal{L}_{identity}$. For our approach, we rely on the original formulation of

$\mathcal{L}_{GAN}$ and $\mathcal{L}_{identity}$, utilizing the L1 norm. We also keep the original formulation of $\mathcal{L}_{cyc}$ for the image domain cycle $\mathcal{X}_I \mapsto \mathcal{X}_L \mapsto \mathcal{X}_I$, but replace the cycle loss for the label domain $\mathcal{X}_L \mapsto \mathcal{X}_I \mapsto \mathcal{X}_L$ by a distance-weighted loss, similar to [1]. This is motivated by the fact, that cell membranes are represented as thin lines and even slight offsets cause large jumps in the L1 loss term, which impedes the training process and results in inaccuracies between membrane positions in the image domain $\mathcal{X}_I$ and label domain $\mathcal{X}_L$. To encourage the generators to preserve exact correspondences between membrane positions, a distance map is generated based on original labels x_L, being minimal at membrane positions and maximal at cell centers and in background regions. This distance map w_{dist} is utilized to weight the L1 distance between x_L and the translated label mask $G_{IL}(G_{LI}(x_L))$, which formulates the cycle-consistency loss as

$$\mathcal{L}_{cyc}(G_{IL}, G_{LI}) = \mathbb{E}_{x_I \sim p_{data}(x_I)}[||G_{LI}(G_{IL}(x_I)) - x_I||_1] \\ + \mathbb{E}_{x_L \sim p_{data}(x_L)}[w_{dist} \cdot ||G_{IL}(G_{LI}(x_L)) - x_L||_1], \tag{1}$$

with p_{data} denoting the data distributions. Instead of using the 3-class representation as input for the generators, only the binary mask of membrane locations is utilized and background and centroid information are omitted. That way, the task of the generators G_{LI} and G_{IL} can be interpreted as a transformation between the reconstructed membrane signal and a degraded representation, captured by the microscope.

3   Experiments

Experiments are based on 2D slices from 3D confocal microscopy image stacks of *A. thqliana* [12], which serve as a baseline data set $\mathcal{D}_{orig}$ for validation. Three additional data sets were generated by the proposed method, showing decreasing abstraction of structures and involving increasing priors of structural appearance. Details of each data set are specified in the following.

3.1   No Correspondence ($\mathcal{D}_{naive}$)

Cell populations in the considered data set roughly resemble a circular structure (Fig. 1). To this end, the first generated data set naively mimics the specimens appearance by generation of a circularly shaped foreground region. Within the foreground region, cell instances are generated by the method described in Sect. 2.1 utilizing the parameter tuple ($n_{points} = 4000, n_{iter} = 100, k = 20$). Subsequently, the cycleGAN approach described in Sect. 2.2 translates the generated labels to the image domain.

3.2   Global Shape Correspondence ($\mathcal{D}_{global}$)

To incorporate more accurate specimen shapes, more realistic foreground regions are estimated from original samples of the image domain $\mathcal{X}_I$, by intensity thresholding and morphological hole filling. Within the foreground region, cell instances are generated as described in Sect. 2.1 utilizing the parameter tuple

$(n_{points} = 4000, n_{iter} = 100, k = 20)$ and subsequently images are synthesized by the cycleGAN approach.

3.3 Local Structure Correspondence ($\mathcal{D}_{local}$)

To further validate our approach, another data set is generated, which skips the label generation step and solely relies on original labels $x_L \in \mathcal{X}_L$. Corresponding images are generated by the cycleGAN approach, which allows to investigate the rate of errors induced by the domain translation. Note that the translation is still trained in an unsupervised fashion, since we do not rely on paired data.

4 Results

The public data set [12] comprises a total of 124 image stacks from 6 different plants with annotations obtained with an automatic method that was manually corrected. Due to the high correlation between neighbouring slices along the z-axis, for each plant we randomly select 200 2D slices at arbitrary z-locations, which reduced the data set $\mathcal{D}_{orig}$ to a total of 1200 2D samples. Each generated data set $\mathcal{D}_{naive}$, $\mathcal{D}_{global}$ and $\mathcal{D}_{local}$, therefore, likewise comprised 200 generated samples per plant.

For evaluation, a three-fold cross-validation was performed, subsequently utilizing four plants for training of the data generation and two for testing. First, the quality of generated images was assessed by considering two different similarity measurements. Second, the generated data sets were utilized for training of a segmentation approach [2] and final segmentation accuracies were compared to those obtained by only using manually annotated data.

4.1 Image Quality Assessment

Similarity between real and fake data was evaluated by the structure similarity measurement (SSIM) and the normalized correlation coefficient (NCC). Following the scheme of the three-fold cross-validation, generated fake images of each test set were compared to the corresponding real image. As the quantitative results in Fig. 2 show, data generated from real labels exhibit the highest degree

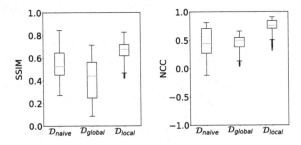

Fig. 2. Boxplots of SSIM and NCC calculated between fake images of each folds test set and the corresponding real images. Red lines indicate the median value and boxes extend from the first to the third quartile. Whiskers show the range of achieved values without considering outliers, which are represented as individual dots. (Color figure online)

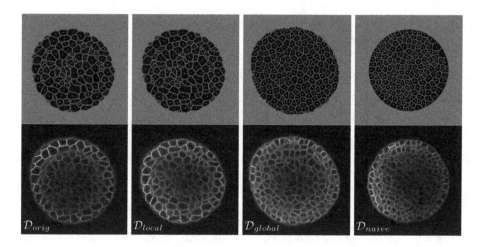

Fig. 3. Multi-class mask of each data set, color coding background in red, membrane positions in blue and centroids in green (first row). The second row shows corresponding images, which are, except for the original data set, generated by the cycleGAN trained on the respectively generated labels. (Color figure online)

of similarity to real data. Small deviations from real labels lead to worse similarity scores, which is attributable to the missing correspondence between exact membrane positions in the real and generated label domain. Qualitative results depicted in Fig. 3, show visually appealing images for all generated data sets. Additionally, it becomes visible that unnatural mask shapes impede the learned correspondences between membrane positions in the label and image domain.

4.2   Training with Synthesized Data

Utilizability of the generated data was assessed by training the segmentation approach presented in [2], which was adapted to work for 2D data. To train more general models, data augmentation was incorporated into the training process,

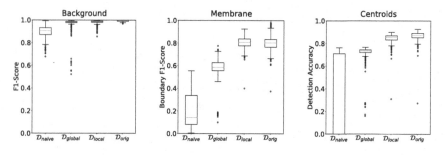

Fig. 4. Scores for segmentation of background, membrane and centroids, obtained by training on the respective domain. Red lines indicate the median value and boxes extend from the first to the third quartile. Whiskers show the range of achieved values without considering outliers, which are represented as individual dots. (Color figure online)

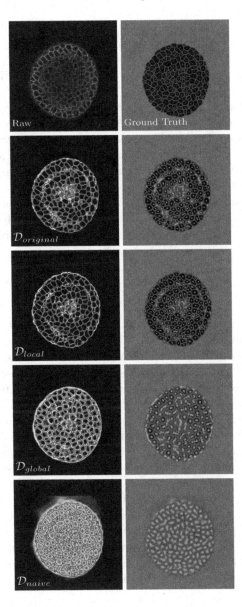

Fig. 5. Right column: multi-class segmentation results for the approach proposed in [2], trained on the respective domain. Left column: membrane predictions are overlayed with the ground truth membrane segmentation (blue). Additionally, the raw image and the ground truth segmentation are shown in the first row. (Color figure online)

which included rotation, flipping, additive Gaussian noise and random intensity scaling in the range $[0.5, 1]$. For validation, one plant of each fold's test set was utilized for training and the second plant for testing and vice versa. This way, it was ensured that overall five plants were used for training (four for data generation and one for segmentation) and the sixth plant was never seen during the training. Note that, computation of segmentation scores for the sixth plant, always considered real samples $x_I \in \mathcal{X}_I$ and manual annotations $x_L \in \mathcal{X}_L$, but no generated data.

Metrics were adapted from [2] and comprised the regular F1-score for background predictions, a boundary F1-score allowing a safety margin of two pixels around each membrane for membrane predictions and a local maximum-based detection accuracy for centroid detection. As a baseline, the segmentation approach was trained on $\mathcal{D}_{orig}$, also deploying the policy to consider one plant for training and one for testing. Quantitative results obtained by utilizing the generated data sets for training are shown in Fig. 4, which analogously to the obtained similarity scores show increasing prediction accuracies of each class with utilization of more realistic data. This is also supported by qualitative results depicted in Fig. 5.

5   Conclusion

In this paper, an approach towards annotation-free segmentation of fluorescently labeled cell membranes was proposed. The concept for label generation demonstrated that even with small correspondences to the real image domain, plausible images could be generated. Training a segmentation approach with generated data disclosed that at least small correspondences between real and generated images had to be included, in order to obtain reliable segmentations. Especially for the naive approach, inaccurate correspondences between membrane positions in the label and image domain impeded the training process and resulted in vague segmentations. Although the loss was modified to penalize offsets of membrane positions in both domains, the offset increased with increasing abstraction of membrane labels. However, the trade-off between less accurate label predictions and the necessity for manual interaction has to be considered, since training without manual labels not only allows to create training data sets of arbitrary size, but additionally completely diminishes the need for tedious and time-consuming manual interactions. In general, the results are a promising first step and we plan to further improve the domain correspondences for the naive approach and to extend the concept to generating realistic 3D data.

References

1. Caliva, F., Iriondo, C., Martinez, A.M., Majumdar, S., Pedoia, V.: Distance map loss penalty term for semantic segmentation. In: International Conference on Medical Imaging with Deep Learning - Extended Abstract Track (2019)
2. Eschweiler, D., Spina, T.V., Choudhury, R.C., Meyerowitz, E., Cunha, A., Stegmaier, J.: CNN-based preprocessing to optimize watershed-based cell segmentation in 3D confocal microscopy images. In: Proceedings of the IEEE International Symposium on Biomedical Imaging, pp. 223–227 (2019)

3. Fernandez, R., et al.: Imaging plant growth in 4D: robust tissue reconstruction and lineaging at cell resolution. Nat. Methods **7**, 547 (2010)
4. Goldsborough, P., Pawlowski, N., Caicedo, J.C., Singh, S., Carpenter, A.E.: Cyto-GAN: generative modeling of cell images. In: bioRxiv, p. 227645 (2017)
5. Majurski, M., et al.: Cell image segmentation using generative adversarial networks, transfer learning, and augmentations. In: Proceedings of the IEEE Conference on Computer Vision and Pattern Recognition Workshops (2019)
6. Mosaliganti, K.R., Noche, R.R., Xiong, F., Swinburne, I.A., Megason, S.G.: ACME: automated cell morphology extractor for comprehensive reconstruction of cell membranes. PLoS Comput. Biol. **8**, e1002780 (2012)
7. Osokin, A., Chessel, A., Carazo-Salas, R.E., Vaggi, F.: GANs for biological image synthesis. In: Proceedings of the IEEE International Conference on Computer Vision, pp. 2233–2242 (2017)
8. Stegmaier, J., et al.: Generating semi-synthetic validation benchmarks for embryomics. In: Proceedings of the IEEE International Symposium on Biomedical Imaging, pp. 684–688 (2016)
9. Stegmaier, J., et al.: Cell segmentation in 3D confocal images using supervoxel merge-forests with CNN-based hypothesis selection. In: Proceedings of the IEEE International Symposium on Biomedical Imaging, pp. 382–386 (2018)
10. Svoboda, D., Kozubek, M., Stejskal, S.: Generation of digital phantoms of cell nuclei and simulation of image formation in 3D image cytometry. Cytometry Part A **75A**(6), 494–509 (2009)
11. Weigert, M., Subramanian, K., Bundschuh, S.T., Myers, E.W., Kreysing, M.: Biobeam - multiplexed wave-optical simulations of light-sheet microscopy. PLoS Comput. Biol. **14**(4), e1006079 (2018)
12. Willis, L., et al.: Cell size and growth regulation in the *Arabidopsis Thaliana* apical stem cell niche. Proc. Natl. Acad. Sci. **113**, 8238–8246 (2016)
13. Zhao, Z., Yang, L., Zheng, H., Guldner, I.H., Zhang, S., Chen, D.Z.: Deep learning based instance segmentation in 3D biomedical images using weak annotation. In: Frangi, A.F., Schnabel, J.A., Davatzikos, C., Alberola-López, C., Fichtinger, G. (eds.) MICCAI 2018. LNCS, vol. 11073, pp. 352–360. Springer, Cham (2018). https://doi.org/10.1007/978-3-030-00937-3_41
14. Zhu, J.Y., Park, T., Isola, P., Efros, A.A.: Unpaired image-to-image translation using cycle-consistent adversarial networks. In: Proceedings of the IEEE International Conference on Computer Vision, pp. 2223–2232 (2017)

Intelligent Image Synthesis to Attack a Segmentation CNN Using Adversarial Learning

Liang Chen[1,2(✉)], Paul Bentley[2], Kensaku Mori[3], Kazunari Misawa[4], Michitaka Fujiwara[5], and Daniel Rueckert[1]

[1] Department of Computing, Imperial College London,
180 Queen's Gate, London SW7 2AZ, UK
liang.chen12@imperial.ac.uk
[2] Department of Medicine, Imperial College London,
Fulham Palace Road, London W6 8RF, UK
[3] Graduate School of Informatics, Nagoya University, Nagoya 464-8603, Japan
[4] The Aichi Cancer Center, Nagoya 464-8681, Japan
[5] Nagoya University Hospital, Nagoya 466-8560, Japan

Abstract. Deep learning approaches based on convolutional neural networks (CNNs) have been successful in solving a number of problems in medical imaging, including image segmentation. In recent years, it has been shown that CNNs are vulnerable to attacks in which the input image is perturbed by relatively small amounts of noise so that the CNN is no longer able to perform a segmentation of the perturbed image with sufficient accuracy. Therefore, exploring methods on how to attack CNN-based models as well as how to defend models against attacks have become a popular topic as this also provides insights into the performance and generalization abilities of CNNs. However, most of the existing work assumes unrealistic attack models, i.e. the resulting attacks were specified in advance. In this paper, we propose a novel approach for generating adversarial examples to attack CNN-based segmentation models for medical images. Our approach has three key features: (1) The generated adversarial examples exhibit anatomical variations (in form of deformations) as well as appearance perturbations; (2) The adversarial examples attack segmentation models so that the Dice scores decrease by a pre-specified amount; (3) The attack is not required to be specified beforehand. We have evaluated our approach on CNN-based approaches for the multi-organ segmentation problem in 2D CT images. We show that the proposed approach can be used to attack different CNN-based segmentation models.

1 Introduction

CNNs have been amongst the most popular model for image classification and segmentation problems thanks to their efficiency and effectiveness in learning representative image features. However, it has been widely reported that even

© Springer Nature Switzerland AG 2019
N. Burgos et al. (Eds.): SASHIMI 2019, LNCS 11827, pp. 90–99, 2019.
https://doi.org/10.1007/978-3-030-32778-1_10

the most well-established CNN models such as the GoogLeNet [14], are vulnerable to almost imperceptible intensity changes to the input images [6]. These small intensity changes can be regarded as adversarial attacks to CNNs. In medical image classification, the adversarial attacks can also fool CNN-based classifiers [3,16]. Therefore, it is important to verify the robustness of CNNs before deploying them into practical use.

The verification of CNNs requires good understanding of the mechanism of adversarial attacks. In this paper, we aim at developing a novel method to generate adversarial examples which are able to attack CNN models for medical image segmentation. Generating adversarial examples to attack semantic image segmentation models is challenging because: (1) Semantic segmentation means assigning a label to each pixel (or voxel) instead of a single label per image as in conventional adversarial attacks typically described in computer vision scenarios. Therefore, attacking a segmentation model is more challenging than attacking a classification model; (2) It is not straightforward to evaluate the success of the attack. A good adversarial example for a classification model results in an incorrect prediction on the whole image while a good adversarial example for a segmentation model does not necessarily lead to an incorrect prediction for every pixel (voxel); (3) Conventional adversarial attacks perturb the image intensity by small amount, however, in medical imaging scenarios deformations are also useful to attack segmentation models. For instance, organs can be present in various configuration in images. Any segmentation model is therefore in principle susceptible to unseen poses or shapes of organs.

Generative adversarial networks (GAN) [5] and variational autoencoders (VAE) [9] are both unsupervised methods that can learn latent feature representations from training images. A GAN learns the latent feature representations implicitly while the VAE learns them explicitly. Training a GAN is difficult due to mode collapse and unreasonable results, e.g. a dog with two heads. In contrast, training a VAE is fairly simple. However, while a GAN can generate realistic images, images generated by a VAE are blurry because of the L2 loss employed during training. Inspired by these observations, we propose to combine the advantages of VAE and GAN to generate realistic and reasonable image deformations and appearance changes so that the transformed images can attack medical segmentation models.

Our main contributions can be summarised as follows: (1) We propose a novel approach to generate adversarial examples to attack the CNN model for abdominal organ segmentation in CT images; (2) We also measure the success of attack by means of observing significant reductions in the Dice score compared to ground truth segmentations; (3) The proposed approach attacking the segmentation model does not require any a-priori specification of particular attacks. In our application, we do not specify any organ which is attacked.

2   Related Work

The work in [4,11], and [19] represent state-of-the-art methods for attacking segmentation models. Fischer et al. [4] proposed to attack segmentation models so that the models cannot segment object in a specified class (e.g. ignoring pedestrians on street). Metzen et al. [11] proposed to generate adversarial examples so that the segmentation model incorrectly segments one cityscape as another one. The adversarial examples generated by these two methods attacked the segmentation models with specified targets, e.g. pedestrians. In contrast, Xie et al. [19] proposed an approach to generate adversarial examples for image semantic segmentation and object detection without attacking targets. However, a random segmentation result should be specified so that the adversaries can be inferred. The adversarial attacks generated by these three methods often appear as pure noise that has no semantic meaning. Therefore, these attacks do not represent real-world situations that can occur in medical imaging applications.

3   Our Approach

We propose a novel end-to-end approach to generate adversarial examples for medical image segmentation scenarios. Formally, I_0 is the original image (H height and W width) and $S_0 \in \mathbb{R}^{H \times W \times (C+1)}$ is its segmentation given a fixed CNN-based segmentation model $f_{seg}(\cdot)$, i.e. $S_0 = f_{seg}(I_0)$. Here C is the number of labels, e.g. the organs of interest. The adversarial attack model allows deformations D and intensity variations V applied to I_0. D is a dense deformation field which is a displacement vector for each pixel (or voxel) while V is a smooth intensity perturbation which can be interpreted, e.g. as a bias field. Therefore, the transformed image after adversarial attack is given by

$$I_{DV} = I_D + V = f_D(I_0, D) + V. \tag{1}$$

Here $f_D(\cdot, \cdot)$ is the function which transforms I_0 to I_D based on D. Figure 1 shows the framework which learns appropriate D and V such that I_{DV} can attack the segmentation model. The whole framework consists of two key components: a CNN model for I_{DV} generation and it's learning algorithm.

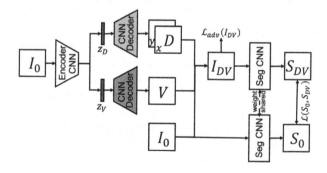

Fig. 1. Overview of the proposed framework. The CNN decoders in blue and green share the same architecture but they do not share weights. (Color figure online)

3.1 Model for Generating Adversarial Attack

The CNN architecture which generates the $\boldsymbol{I}_{DV}$ is similar to a multi-task VAE. First, $\boldsymbol{I}_0$ is processed by an encoding CNN resulting in several feature maps which are then used to learn a latent feature representation $\boldsymbol{z}_D \sim \mathcal{N}(\boldsymbol{\mu}_D, \boldsymbol{\sigma}_D^2)$ and $\boldsymbol{z}_V \sim \mathcal{N}(\boldsymbol{\mu}_V, \boldsymbol{\sigma}_V^2)$. $\boldsymbol{z}_D$ and $\boldsymbol{z}_V$ are then reconstructed to dense deformation field $\boldsymbol{D}$ and dense intensity variation $\boldsymbol{V}$ by two CNN decoders, respectively. The two decoding CNNs share the same architecture but they do not share weights. Learning $\boldsymbol{z}_D$ and $\boldsymbol{z}_V$ explicitly ensures the $\boldsymbol{I}_{DV}$ looks reasonable.

The dense deformation $\boldsymbol{D}$ consists of two channels of feature maps $\boldsymbol{D}_x$ and $\boldsymbol{D}_y$, representing pixel position changes in horizontal and vertical directions (i.e. x and y axis). In addition, we propose to limit the norm of $\boldsymbol{D}$ and $\boldsymbol{V}$ so that it is difficult to be perceived by human observers. To this end, the following to regularization terms are used:

$$\mathcal{L}(\boldsymbol{D}) = \lambda_D \|\boldsymbol{D}\|_2^2; \quad \mathcal{L}(\boldsymbol{V}) = \lambda_V \|\boldsymbol{V}\|_2^2. \tag{2}$$

λ_D and λ_V are two fixed hyper-parameters. The regularization ensures the smoothness of the deformation field $\boldsymbol{D}$ and intensity variation $\boldsymbol{V}$.

Each branch of the CNNs generating $\boldsymbol{I}_{DV}$ is different from a VAE since the input and output of the CNN are not the same. In fact, it is an image-to-image CNN and we can sample the learned latent space to generate multiple instances $\boldsymbol{D}$s and $\boldsymbol{V}$s. This idea is similar to the one proposed in [10] where a latent space was learned to sample multiple realistic image segmentations.

3.2 Learning

Since the ground truth of $\boldsymbol{D}$, $\boldsymbol{V}$, and $\boldsymbol{I}_{DV}$ are not available, it is not possible to learn the parameters of the encoding and decoding CNN in a explicit supervised manner. To address this problem, we propose to learn the parameters implicitly based on two conditions: First, we assume that $\boldsymbol{I}_{DV}$ should look realistic compared with $\boldsymbol{I}_0$. Secondly we assume that the accuracy of the segmentation $\boldsymbol{S}_{DV}$ should decreases significantly compared with $\boldsymbol{S}_0$. This decrease can be measured in terms of a reduction of Dice score.

An adversarial learning method is employed to ensure the $\boldsymbol{I}_{DV}$ looks realistic compared with $\boldsymbol{I}_0$. To this end, the $\boldsymbol{I}_{DV}$ generating CNN is regarded as a generator CNN, i.e. $\boldsymbol{I}_{DV} = f_{gen}(\boldsymbol{I}_0)$. An additional discriminator CNN $f_{disc}(\cdot)$ is used to predict the realism of $\boldsymbol{I}_{DV}$ compared with $\boldsymbol{I}_0$ [8]. Adversarial training $f_{gen}(\cdot)$ and $f_{disc}(\cdot)$ results in realistic $\boldsymbol{I}_{DV}$. We adopt the Wasserstein GAN (WGAN) [1] loss function during the adversarial training. Formally,

$$\begin{aligned} \mathcal{L}_{adv}^{gen} &= f_{disc}(\boldsymbol{I}_0) - f_{disc}(\boldsymbol{I}_{DV}), \\ \mathcal{L}_{adv}^{disc} &= f_{disc}(\boldsymbol{I}_{DV}) - f_{disc}(\boldsymbol{I}_0). \end{aligned} \tag{3}$$

The goal of this work is to generate $\boldsymbol{I}_{DV}$ which is able to attack a given segmentation CNN model, e.g. a U-Net [13]. This means that the segmentation results $\boldsymbol{S}_0$ and $\boldsymbol{S}_{DV}$ are different. Here $\boldsymbol{S}_{DV} = f_{seg}(\boldsymbol{I}_{DV})$. When training $f_{seg}(\cdot)$, we use cross-entropy as the loss function between S_0 and the ground truth S_{GT}, i.e. $f_{xent}(S_0, S_{GT}) = -\sum_{c=0}^{C} S_{GT}(c) \log(S_0(c))$. This leads to satisfactory S_0. To constrain the difference between S_0 and S_{DV}, we propose to use the following loss function:

$$\mathcal{L}(S_0, S_{DV}) = (\xi - f_{xent}^M(S_0, S_{DV}))^2. \tag{4}$$

Here ξ is a hyper-parameter which controls the difference between S_0 and S_{DV}. If $\xi = 0$, then S_{DV} tends to be similar to S_0 so that D and V tend to be zero. In contrast, if ξ is a very large number, then the norm of D and V are large that the discriminator CNN is difficult to fool. As such, the training process is likely to collapse. Therefore, ξ should be within a proper range. In addition, we propose to mask the standard cross-entropy function so that the ROI of organs of interest is emphasized. Specifically, the masked cross-entropy function is

$$f_{xent}^M(S_{DV}, S_0) = -\sum_{c=1}^{C} S_0(c) * \sum_{c=0}^{C} S_0(c) \log(S_{DV}(c)). \tag{5}$$

Here, $M = \sum_{c=1}^{C} S_0(c)$ is the mask highlighting the organs of interest and $*$ is the element-wise product.

In summary, the loss functions of the whole framework are:

$$\begin{aligned} \mathcal{L}^{gen} &= \mathcal{L}_{adv}^{gen} + \mathcal{L}(S_0, S_{DV}) + \mathcal{L}(D) + \mathcal{L}(V), \\ \mathcal{L}^{disc} &= \mathcal{L}_{adv}^{disc}. \end{aligned} \tag{6}$$

3.3 Implementation Details

In this paper, CNNs are implemented using Tensorflow. The adversarial learning is optimised using the RMSProp algorithm [17]. The decay is 0.9 and $\epsilon = 10^{-10}$. We use the fixed learning rate of 10^{-4} for both generator and discriminator CNNs. Batch normalization technique [7] is used after convolutions. A leaky rectified linear unit (LReLU) is used as the nonlinear activation function to ease the adversarial training with $\alpha = 0.2$. λ_D and λ_V are set as 0.1 and 0.01, respectively.

4 Experiments and Results

Experiments were performed on a abdominal CT dataset with multiple organs manually annotated by human experts. The image acquisition details and the involved patient demographics can be found in [18]. The dataset consists of 150 subjects and for each subject the annotated organs include the pancreas, the kidneys, the liver, and the spleen. The dataset was randomly split into a training set, a validation set, and a testing set, which have 60, 15, and 75 subjects respectively. The voxel intensities of each subject were normalized to zero mean and unit standard deviation.

We trained a standard U-Net [13] to segment all abdominal organs. Due to limitations with GPU memory, the U-Net is based on 2D image, rather than 3D volumes. Following [2], the U-Net was trained on image patches and tested on image slices. The trained U-Net was used as the fixed CNN in this work to be subjected by adversarial attacks.

The Dice score was used to assess the segmentation quality for each organ. We define a 30% decrease on the Dice score of an organ as a successful attack. Similar to [12, 15], we compute the perceptibility p of the adversarial perturbation $r = I_{DV} - I_0$ by

$$p = \frac{1}{HW} \sum_{i,j} |r_{i,j}|. \tag{7}$$

p is the similarity of the real image to the synthetic image. The smaller the value of p is, the less likely the adversarial perturbation is perceived by human observers.

4.1 Adversarial Examples

By sampling the learned latent spaces, the deformation D and the intensity variation V are generated and therefore realistic adversarial examples are obtained. Figure 2 shows two such examples. Thanks to the regularization imposed on D and V, both are smooth and difficult to recognise by humans. However, the derived adversarial examples attack the U-Net successfully. More examples are shown in Fig. 3.

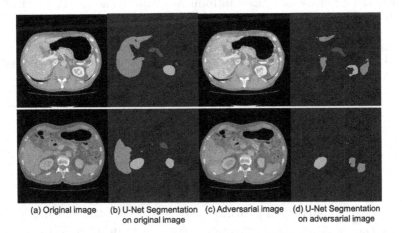

(a) Original image   (b) U-Net Segmentation   (c) Adversarial image   (d) U-Net Segmentation
on original image   on adversarial image

Fig. 2. Example CT abdominal image, the resulting U-Net segmentation, the generated adversarial CT images using the proposed method, and the resulting U-Net segmentation of the adversarial images. In the segmentations, the pancreas, the kidneys, the liver, and the spleen are depicted in blue, green, orange, and red, respectively. In this case, $\xi = 2.0$. (Color figure online)

4.2   Attacking the Segmentation Model

Table 1 shows the segmentation results of the standard U-Net on multiple organs. The aforementioned success of the attacking model results in a 30% decrease in terms of Dice score on every organ. We also listed this borderline of Dice score in Table 1. In the proposed attack approach, ξ is an important hyper-parameter deciding the success of attacking the U-Net. ξ ranging from 0.5 to 3.0 was tested and the results are shown in Table 1. The larger the ξ is, the more the Dice scores decrease and the larger the perceptibility is. Using $\xi \geq 2.0$, the U-Net can be attacked successfully on all organs.

In terms of different organs, the segmentations on the pancreas and the kidneys are more difficult to be attacked compared to segmentations on the liver and the spleen. Specifically, the segmentations on the pancreas and the kidneys can be attacked when $\xi \geq 2.0$ while the segmentations on the liver and the spleen can be attacked when $\xi \geq 1.0$.

The proposed adversarial examples feature both deformations D and intensity variations V. We studied the effect of D and V individually when $\xi = 2.0$. The results are reported in Table 1. For the kidneys, the deformation changes lead to more decrease of the Dice scores while on the other organs, the intensity variance has more impact on attacking the U-Net model. This means that the segmentation model is more sensitive to the intensity variance. The abdominal organs naturally vary in terms of pose on 2D image slices in the training set. Therefore, small deformations do not significantly decrease the Dice scores. In contrast, the intensity variations introduces shadows and artefacts which are likely to influence the segmentation CNN.

Table 1. Abdominal organ segmentation comparison among different configurations in terms of the Dice score (%)

	Dice				p
	Pancreas	Kidneys	Liver	Spleen	
U-Net	80.07	94.74	94.71	94.76	–
U-Net 30% decrease	56.05	66.32	66.30	66.33	–
I_{DV} on U-Net ($\xi = 0.5$)	74.77	93.88	89.81	81.87	0.061
I_{DV} on U-Net ($\xi = 1.0$)	70.66	90.06	59.51	37.12	0.060
I_{DV} on U-Net ($\xi = 1.5$)	64.25	66.97	26.45	35.81	0.075
I_{DV} on U-Net ($\xi = 2.0$)	53.59	60.07	11.19	17.21	0.074
I_{DV} on U-Net ($\xi = 2.5$)	40.57	45.47	9.16	17.60	0.084
I_{DV} on U-Net ($\xi = 3.0$)	31.49	43.43	5.82	26.58	0.085
I_D on U-Net ($\xi = 2.0$)	70.46	82.04	75.06	70.47	0.056
I_V on U-Net ($\xi = 2.0$)	68.15	88.25	50.05	46.94	0.061

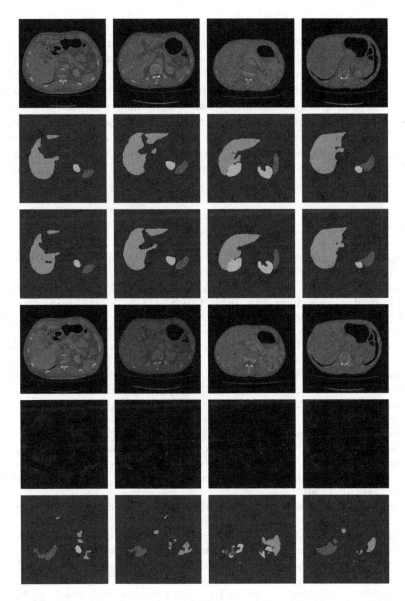

Fig. 3. Some additional visual results of the proposed method. Each column represents an individual case. $I_0, S_{GT}, S_0, I_{DV}, V, S_{DV}$ are shown from the top row to the bottom row

5 Discussion and Conclusion

In this paper, we have proposed a novel approach to generate adversarial examples to attack an existing CNN model for medical image segmentation. The generated adversarial examples include geometrical deformations to model anatomical variations as well as intensity variation which model appearance variations. These examples attack CNN-based segmentation models such as a U-Net [13] by decreasing the Dice score by a pre-specified amount. The training process is end-to-end without any predefined requirements. In fact, it can be replaced by any other CNN-based models. In the future, we will investigate the use of the proposed approach to generate additional training images so that the segmentation model can be more robust and defend attacks. In addition, the proposed approach can be used to verify if an CNN model is robust or not. Specifically, our approach can generate adversarial examples for the CNN model. If the adversarial examples are reasonable and realistic, then the CNN model is not robust enough.

References

1. Arjovsky, M., Chintala, S., Bottou, L.: Wasserstein generative adversarial networks. In: ICML, pp. 214–223 (2017)
2. Chen, L., Bentley, P., Mori, K., Misawa, K., Fujiwara, M., Rueckert, D.: DRINet for medical image segmentation. IEEE TMI **37**(11), 2453–2462 (2018)
3. Finlayson, S.G., Kohane, I.S., Beam, A.L.: Adversarial attacks against medical deep learning systems. arXiv preprint arXiv:1804.05296 (2018)
4. Fischer, V., Kumar, M.C., Metzen, J.H., Brox, T.: Adversarial examples for semantic image segmentation. arXiv preprint arXiv:1703.01101 (2017)
5. Goodfellow, I., et al.: Generative adversarial nets. In: NIPS, pp. 2672–2680 (2014)
6. Goodfellow, I.J., Shlens, J., Szegedy, C.: Explaining and harnessing adversarial examples. In: ICLR (2015)
7. Ioffe, S., Szegedy, C.: Batch normalization: accelerating deep network training by reducing internal covariate shift. In: ICML, pp. 448–456 (2015)
8. Jolicoeur-Martineau, A.: The relativistic discriminator: a key element missing from standard GAN. arXiv preprint arXiv:1807.00734 (2018)
9. Kingma, D.P., Welling, M.: Auto-encoding variational Bayes. arXiv preprint arXiv:1312.6114 (2013)
10. Kohl, S., et al.: A probabilistic U-Net for segmentation of ambiguous images. In: NIPS, pp. 6965–6975 (2018)
11. Metzen, J.H., Kumar, M.C., Brox, T., Fischer, V.: Universal adversarial perturbations against semantic image segmentation. In: ICCV, pp. 2755–2764 (2017)
12. Nguyen, A., Yosinski, J., Clune, J.: Deep neural networks are easily fooled: high confidence predictions for unrecognizable images. In: CVPR, pp. 427–436 (2015)
13. Ronneberger, O., Fischer, P., Brox, T.: U-Net: convolutional networks for biomedical image segmentation. In: Navab, N., Hornegger, J., Wells, W.M., Frangi, A.F. (eds.) MICCAI 2015. LNCS, vol. 9351, pp. 234–241. Springer, Cham (2015). https://doi.org/10.1007/978-3-319-24574-4_28
14. Szegedy, C., et al.: Going deeper with convolutions. In: CVPR, pp. 1–9 (2015)
15. Szegedy, C., et al.: Intriguing properties of neural networks. In: ICLR (2014)
16. Asgari Taghanaki, S., Das, A., Hamarneh, G.: Vulnerability analysis of chest X-Ray image classification against adversarial attacks. In: Stoyanov, D., et al. (eds.) MLCN/DLF/IMIMIC -2018. LNCS, vol. 11038, pp. 87–94. Springer, Cham (2018). https://doi.org/10.1007/978-3-030-02628-8_10

17. Tieleman, T., Hinton, G.: Lecture 6.5-RMSProp: divide the gradient by a running average of its recent magnitude. COURSERA: Neural Netw. Mach. Learn. **4**(2), 26–31 (2012)
18. Tong, T., et al.: Discriminative dictionary learning for abdominal multi-organ segmentation. Med. Image Anal. **23**(1), 92–104 (2015)
19. Xie, C., Wang, J., Zhang, Z., Zhou, Y., Xie, L., Yuille, A.: Adversarial examples for semantic segmentation and object detection. In: ICCV, pp. 1369–1378 (2017)

Physics-Informed Brain MRI Segmentation

Pedro Borges[1,2(✉)], Carole Sudre[1,2,3], Thomas Varsavsky[1,2], David Thomas[3], Ivana Drobnjak[1], Sebastien Ourselin[2], and M. Jorge Cardoso[2]

[1] Department of Medical Physics and Biomedical Engineering, UCL, London, UK
p.borges.17@ucl.ac.uk
[2] School of Biomedical Engineering and Imaging Sciences, KCL, London, UK
[3] Dementia Research Centre, UCL, London, UK

Abstract. Magnetic Resonance Imaging (MRI) is one of the most flexible and powerful medical imaging modalities. This flexibility does however come at a cost; MRI images acquired at different sites and with different parameters exhibit significant differences in contrast and tissue appearance, resulting in downstream issues when quantifying brain anatomy or the presence of pathology. In this work, we propose to combine multiparametric MRI-based static-equation sequence simulations with segmentation convolutional neural networks (CNN), to make these networks robust to variations in acquisition parameters. Results demonstrate that, when given both the image and their associated physics acquisition parameters, CNNs can produce segmentations that exhibit robustness to acquisition variations. We also show that the proposed physics-informed methods can be used to bridge multi-centre and longitudinal imaging studies where imaging acquisition varies across a site or in time.

Keywords: MRI · Harmonization · Deep learning

1 Introduction

Magnetic Resonance Imaging (MRI) is a widespread, non-invasive, non-ionizing medical imaging technique. It is capable of imaging any part of the body to produce three dimensional anatomical and functional reconstructions, excelling at soft tissue contrast. MRI is therefore aptly suited for looking at pathological changes in the brain, such as tissue atrophy or lesions. However, large scale studies that rely on multiple scanners from different manufacturers suffer from site and hardware-dependent variabilities in the acquired data [13]. Without means to account for these differences, this variability impacts our ability to conduct multi-centre analyses and extract meaningful and reproducible biomarkers [6]. Further challenges are encountered in longitudinal studies since scanner and sequence protocol changes cause inconsistencies in patient imaging that make disease evolution impossible to quantify.

N. Burgos et al. (Eds.): SASHIMI 2019, LNCS 11827, pp. 100–109, 2019.
https://doi.org/10.1007/978-3-030-32778-1_11

One issue caused by the non-quantitative nature of MRI images is that algorithms are often unable to deal with different sequence parameters. For example, if MR images are acquired with small differences in acquisition, segmentation algorithms often produce disparate results, exhibiting apparent growth/shrinkage of regions of interest [4]: this is caused by signal intensity changes that depend on the tissue. Dementia is an example of a condition in which MR imaging biomarkers such as cortical atrophy or hippocampal volume can be used for the diagnosis of the condition. Due to the difficulty in disentangling imaging physics and underlying anatomy, even trained clinicians may fail to account for protocol differences. This is explained by the fact that the information available to the users is limited to voxel intensities, which are unreliable, and *a priori* knowledge of brain morphology, which is not subject-specific.

Current methods to mitigate these effects are cumbersome and imperfect. They normally rely on either a per-site analysis followed by a joint meta-analysis [5] or the use of statistical models with linear covariates [1], which provide computationally efficient yet often inaccurate means of standardization. When attempted, correction for scanning variability can either be made at the tissue-class or the voxel level. The former may be less robust due to the lack of granularity whilst the latter is highly susceptible to errors induced by the required registration to a group-wise space.

Gaining robustness to pulse sequences has been investigated in [10] implicitly, where parameter estimation combined with simulation as an augmentation to a segmentation task is employed. Note however that parameters are bulk-assigned to segmentation maps and that the segmentation network is not physics aware.

This work aims to address the issue of acquisition-induced biomarker extraction variability (resulting from imprecise segmentations) through the use of a novel physics-informed convolutional neural network, where segmentation is used as a pretext task. Parametric tissue maps, together with sequence simulating models, are used to generate realistic samples as if they were acquired with different physics parameters. The importance of MRI sequence simulators is crucial here — they can be used to train machine learning algorithms to learn the features of scanners or sequence parameters without having to expend a vast amount of resources to acquire real data, while realistically reproducing an MRI scan. For computational reasons, we propose to use a static equation-based simulation approach, which makes use of simplified imaging equations to most efficiently generate sufficiently large and varied datasets required for this undertaking. By providing both simulated samples and associated physics parameters as training data for a neural network, we can demonstrate that these networks can produce segmentations that are robust to MRI physics variations because they are explicitly learning how the physics interacts with image contrast.

2   Methodology

Here we describe how physics-based image synthesis is combined with the proposed physics-informed architecture to achieve more consistent segmentations.

2.1   MRI Simulation Methods

The signal intensity obtained in MR images results from the non-linear interaction between tissue properties and parameters associated with a specific acquisition sequence. In this work, we use a simplified, yet robust, simulation model by which static singular equations are employed for each simulated sequence previously employed by [9]. These equations take as input the tissue properties and MR sequence parameters and produce an image of the corresponding sequence. The assumption that signal intensity at any given voxel is based on tissue, sequence, and scanner properties is made here. Contrarily to more complex MR simulators, the proposed model assumes the signal does not change in time, i.e. the model described as 'static'. In this work, we focus on two widely used gradient echo T1-weighted sequences, namely 3D spoiled Gradient echo (SPGR) and 3D magnetization prepared gradient echo (MPRAGE). For both sequences, $PD(x)$, $T_1(x)$ and $T_2^*(x)$ are respectively the proton density, T_1 value and T_2^* value of the tissue at position x, θ is the sequence flip angle, TR the relaxation time and TE the echo time. For the SPGR sequence, the static equation derived by Jog *et al.* [9] expresses the voxel intensity $b_S(x)$ at position x as

$$b_S(x) = G_S PD(x) sin\theta \frac{1 - e^{-\frac{TR}{T_1(x)}}}{1 - \cos\theta e^{-\frac{TR}{T_1(x)}}} e^{-\frac{TE}{T_2^*(x)}}, \tag{1}$$

where G_S is the scanner gain. Similarly, the static equation for MPRAGE sequences describes the intensity $b_M(x)$ at position x as

$$b_M(x) = G_M PD(x) \left(1 - \frac{2e^{\frac{-TI}{T_1(x)}}}{1 + e^{\frac{-(TI+TD+\tau)}{T_1(x)}}} \right), \tag{2}$$

where G_M is the scanner gain, TD the delay time, and τ the slice imaging time.

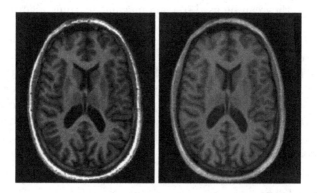

Fig. 1. Left: Middle axial slice of simulated MPRAGE volume with TI = 600 ms. Right: Middle axial slice of simulated MPRAGE volume with TI = 1200 ms. Note the difference in tissue contrasts, particularly between white and cortical grey matter.

A variable inversion time (TI) results in images of differing contrasts owing to the non-linear signal scaling of the different tissue types. Figure 1 illustrates the phenomenon, showcasing two axial slices of MPRAGE simulations with TIs of 800 and 1200 ms, respectively, simulated from the same set of parametric maps.

2.2 Physics-Aware CNNs for Image Segmentation

We propose to inject the sequence parameters of an input image in a CNN network by the addition of a fully connected layer. Since a strong correlation between segmentation volumes and parameter choice can be observed, we expect the introduction of the physics parameters to allow such a network to account for the physics induced appearance variability and attain a more consistent, unmarred segmentation.

2.3 Network Architecture

We used the 3D U-Net architecture as described in [3] as a starting point for the proposed physics injected network. Our proposed architecture (Fig. 2) adds an adjacent branch (physics branch), boasting two fully connected layers of ten neurons each which have as input an N-dimensional vector. This vector consists of the variable physics parameters used to generate the image to be segmented, as well as negative exponentiation of said parameters. The latter is included as a means of making the network privy to the underlying simulation process. This branch is connected to the network via a concatenation operation that broadcasts the branch's output as additional channels immediately following the final shortcut connection of the base 3D U-Net architecture.

3   Experiments

3.1   Creation of Physics-Based Gold Standard Segmentation

It is important to reiterate the primary goal of this work, which is to mitigate the detrimental effects of imaging parameter choices on the consistency of MRI

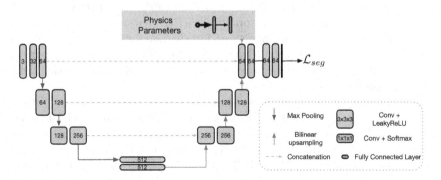

Fig. 2. Diagramatic representation of the proposed network. The novel contribution is primarily the pink box (physics-aware subnet) and the simulation framework used to train the model. (Color figure online)

image segmentations. As such, we are primarily concerned with achieving segmentations that are consistent across acquisitions, more so than approaching a hypothetical 'ground truth' segmentation. With this in mind, and as proper ground truth tissue segmentations are 'illusory' in brain imaging (i.e. humans often disagree, and image resolution is insufficient), we propose to create a gold standard reference segmentation that is consistent and stable across subjects, i.e. one that is precise, concordant and systematic, but not necessarily accurate.

To achieve this, and owing to the T1-W nature of the simulations we propose a "Physics Gold Standard", whereby we make use of the quantitative R_1 maps for this purpose. By assuming that tissues can be parameterised by normal distributions, with mean and standard deviations equivalent to literature R_1 values, we can generate segmentation maps directly from quantitative acquisitions, thereby being largely independent of acquisition physics. Because there can be some significant variation in quantitative maps, we opt to use parameters derived from works whose multiparametric map creation protocol most resembles our own, with an increased standard deviation to account for some additional variability. To this end, the R_1 values we choose are 0.683 ± 0.080 ms for grey matter, 1.036 ± 0.080 ms for white matter, taken from [15]. We note that [15] do not quote values for CSF, but as per [12] which cites multiple other studies on this matter, the R_1 values for CSF are largely independent of acquisition parameters. Due to this, and the fact that we only focus on grey and white matter segmentation consistency in this work, we opt to model our normal CSF distribution with 0.240 ± 0.03 ms, one of the cited values that most closely matched the R_1 CSF measurements in our maps. Using this "Physics Gold Standard" we can model each tissue in a probabilistic, and more anatomically grounded, manner without having to concern ourselves with the inherent bias that would be associated with choosing a more typical "ground truth".

3.2 Datasets

27 multiparametric volumes from an early onset Alzheimer's disease dataset containing both patients and controls were used for simulation. The maps consist of R_1 (longitudinal magnetisation relaxation rate), R_2^* (effective transverse magnetisation relaxation rate), proton density (PD), and magnetisation transfer (MT). We make use of the former three for the simulations. These maps are acquired via three 3D multi-echo FLASH (fast low angle shot) acquisitions further described in [8]. All subjects were rigidly registered to MNI space before their use in simulations.

As a real-world data example, we used a subset of the SABRE dataset consisting of data from 22 subjects drawn from an elderly population with high cardiovascular risk factors, where each subject was imaged within the same scanning session using two different T1-W MPRAGE protocols and one Turbo Spin-Echo protocol. We use only the paired MPRAGE images in this work. Mid-space (so as not to bias the registration towards either acquisition protocol) intra-subject registrations are carried out to resample these images to be 1 mm isotropic.

Table 1. Mean dice scores of GIF, base 3D U-Net and 3D U-Net-Physics methods on segmentation task across inference subjects. All dice scores are estimated against a Physics Gold Standard.

Experiments	Sequences			
	MPRAGE		SPGR	
	GM	WM	GM	WM
GIF	0.851 ± 0.020	0.919 ± 0.009	0.916 ± 0.010	0.847 ± 0.018
Base	0.904 ± 0.024	0.943 ± 0.012	0.946 ± 0.017	0.902 ± 0.021
Physics	0.910 ± 0.017	0.948 ± 0.009	0.948 ± 0.019	0.907 ± 0.015

3.3 Simulation Experiment and Results

For each of the 27 subjects acquired with a multiparametric acquisition, we simulated 121 MPRAGE volumes with TIs between 600 and 1200 ms (5 ms increments) with constant TD of 600 ms and constant τ of 10 ms. These values were chosen by extending the optimised range of 900–1200 ms found in [14]. Similarly, 121 SPGR volumes were simulated per subject sampling randomly from the parameter space spanning TR between 15 and 100 ms, TE between 4 and 10 ms, and FA between 15 and 75°. These values were chosen according to the typical values explored in [9] for SPGR sequences. For each subject, a single "Physics Gold Standard" segmentation was used across the associated synthesized images.

3.4 Robustness to Acquisition Parameters

We train our network on 3D $96 \times 96 \times 96$ randomly sampled from the simulated volumes. For the MPRAGE volumes, TI and e^{-TI} are passed as a vector into the physics branch while for SPGR volumes a vector containing TR, TE, FA, e^{-TR}, e^{-TE}, and $sin(FA)$ is passed as input to the physics branch. Subjects were randomly split between training (2420 simulated volumes over 19 subjects), validation (242 simulated volumes over two subjects) and testing (726 simulated volumes over six subjects). Networks were trained until convergence, as defined per performance on the validation set when over 1000 iterations have elapsed without decreases in the loss (a probabilistic version of the dice loss [11]), using NiftyNet [7], a deep learning framework designed for medical imaging.

In a first instance, we compare the performance of 3D U-Net-Physics with that of base 3D U-Net (trained simply by excluding the physics branch), as well as GIF [2], a segmentation software based on geodesical information flows. Segmentation stability for the two tissue classes is assessed via measures of the coefficient of variability within the set of synthesized data for each test subject. Results, presented in Table 2 show that for MPRAGE simulation, the model enhanced with the Physics branch provides more stable volume estimates for the two tissue classes. Table 1 shows the dice scores for the segmentations compared to the "Physics Gold Standard". It is apparent that "accuracy"-wise all

Table 2. Mean coefficients of variability resulting from GIF, 3D U-Net and 3D U-Net-Physics methods on segmentation task across inference subjects

Experiments	Sequences			
	MPRAGE		SPGR	
	GM	WM	GM	WM
GIF	0.00619	0.00783	**0.00114**	0.00091
Base	0.00332	0.01491	0.00531	0.00160
Physics	**0.00244**	**0.00405**	0.00425	**0.00083**

methods perform similarly. A sign-rank test is carried out to calculate the p-value of the Physics and Base method dices, resulting in p <0.0001, indicating the Physics model's higher performance is statistically significant. The larger gap in performance between the CNN and GIF methods can likely be attributed to differences exhibited between our "Physics Gold Standard" and more typical segmentation ground truths, the latter being closer to what GIF might output. For a single subject, we plot in Fig. 3 the resulting variations in extracted volumes for a range of TI compared to the standard obtained at 900 ms for WM (left) and GM (right). The introduction of the physics branch to the model appears to noticeably reduce the variability observed when using a non-physics aware network.

3.5   Application to a Data Bridging Study

MRI acquisitions are often updated due to hardware or sequence changes, harming our ability to perform ongoing clinical research studies and to compare

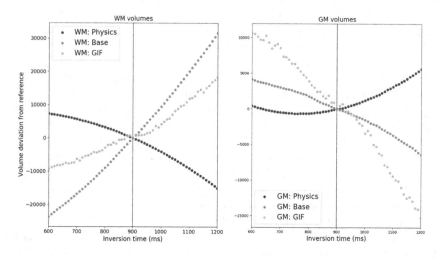

Fig. 3. Comparing the (left) WM and (right) GM volume consistency for simulated data within the 600–1200 TI range over three methods (GIF, Baseline, Physics). Volumes are presented as a deviation from the volume at TI = 900 ms.

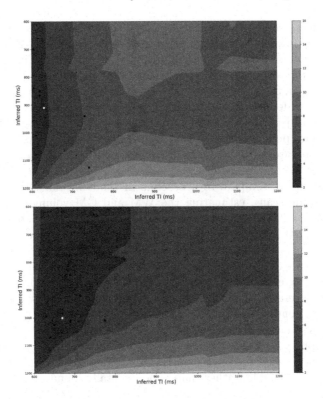

Fig. 4. Top: GM contour of mean percent volume differences across a "training" (12 subjects) subset of SABRE paired dataset. Bottom: WM contour of mean percent volume differences across a "training" (12 subjects) subset of SABRE paired dataset. Black points: Ideal params for each of 10 "test" subjects. White point: Point of volume pair minimisation for "training" subjects.

patients longitudinally. This experiment aims to test if the proposed method could be used to compensate for acquisition parameter updates from an image segmentation biomarker. To do this, we use the 3D-UNet-Physics network trained in the previous section and applied it to the Bridge SABRE dataset, where each subject has a pre and a post parameter update MRI acquisition. Despite images being acquired back-to-back, these images exhibit significant differences owing to differing scanning protocols. As MRI acquisition parameters were not available for this data, we experimentally found an optimal TI parameter that, if applied to the pre-update and post-update acquisition parameters, would make the segmentations between those as close as possible. To achieve this, we partitioned the data into two sets, a "training" set with 12 image pairs, and a "test" set with 10 image pairs. We segment all training set pairs with different hypothetical TI values (i.e. run inference on our physics informed network for each image 121 times, passing a different value of TI from the 600–1200 ms TI range at each pass), and plot the similarity (volume-wise) between TI pairs in Fig. 4 as a contour. This plot shows us how the similarity between GM and WM between the pairs changes according to the TI passed at inference to segment the images. The white point in the figure represents the pre/post TI pair that minimizes the volume difference between training set examples. Finally, we apply this TI parameter pair to the hold-out test set and test if the output segmentations were bridged. Similarly to the white point, the black points indicate the TI pairing that provided the smallest difference in tissue segmentation volumes for each of the 10 subjects. Qualitatively, we observe clustering of these black points around the white point, indicating that this choice of parameters generalizes to the holdout standardization subjects, lending credence to the model's ability to account for the imaging process.

To quantitatively compare to a baseline method, we ran GIF on both pre and post upgrade scans, estimating the WM and GM volumes for each subject - here denoted GIF-Uncorrected. We then find a linear mapping between pre- and post-sequence upgrade volumes on the training set as a form of correction/bridging, and apply it to the hold-out test set - here denoted GIF-Corrected. GIF-Uncorrected exhibits a volumetric difference over tissues of 5%. We found that the linear correction method applied to GIF resulted in a mean volumetric segmentation difference of 3% over tissues. When using the physics model (i.e. choosing the aforementioned ideal parameter pairs denoted by the white point in Fig. 4), this value was found to be 2%. While the differences do not seem large, any improvements are beneficial for the sample size for a hypothetical trial. Consistency could have been potentially improved further if true physics parameters were available, rather than experimentally found.

4   Discussion and Conclusions

This work aimed to address the problem of imaging induced variability in biomarker extraction by constructing networks that are privy to those imaging parameter choices. We show that, for MPRAGE-type sequences, our method outperforms its alternatives, particularly with regards to grey matter. For SPGR we note that performance is more tissue dependent, with small, but significant, decreases in grey matter segmentation consistency compared to competing methods but presenting improvements in white matter consistency. Despite this, it is worth noting that our physics informed network always outperforms its base counterpart, lending credence to the notion that these external parameters can always be leveraged towards some gain in segmentation consistency.

Further work is needed to ascertain the ideal architectural setup for passing external parameters. While the proposed construction performs well for MPRAGE sequences, the results suggest that this might not be the case for others, especially if multiple parameters are involved: The network may require a greater capacity to leverage the additional information.

Results on real data show that the proposed method improved the consistency of estimated volumes, even when the acquisition parameters were found experimentally. Future work will test the proposed method on a more diverse range of protocols and will apply it to larger bridge studies where significant improvements stand to be made.

Acknowledgements. We gratefully acknowledge the support of NVIDIA Corporation with the donation of one Titan V. This project has received funding from Welcome Flagship Programme (WT213038/Z/18/Z) and Welcome EPSRC CME (WT203148/Z/16/Z).

References

1. Ashburner, J., et al.: Voxel-based morphometry—the methods. NeuroImage **11**(6), 805–821 (2000)
2. Cardoso, M.J., et al.: Geodesic information flows: spatially-variant graphs and their application to segmentation and fusion. IEEE Trans. Med. Imaging **34**(9), 1976–1988 (2015)
3. Çiçek, Ö., Abdulkadir, A., Lienkamp, S.S., Brox, T., Ronneberger, O.: 3D U-Net: learning dense volumetric segmentation from sparse annotation. In: Ourselin, S., Joskowicz, L., Sabuncu, M.R., Unal, G., Wells, W. (eds.) MICCAI 2016. LNCS, vol. 9901, pp. 424–432. Springer, Cham (2016). https://doi.org/10.1007/978-3-319-46723-8_49
4. Clark, K.A., et al.: Impact of acquisition protocols and processing streams on tissue segmentation of T1 weighted MR images. Neuroimage **29**(1), 185–202 (2006)
5. van Erp, T.G.M., et al.: Subcortical brain volume abnormalities in 2028 individuals with schizophrenia and 2540 healthy controls via the ENIGMA consortium. Mol. Psychiatry **21**(4), 547–553 (2015)
6. Frisoni, G.B., et al.: Strategic roadmap for an early diagnosis of alzheimers disease based on biomarkers. Lancet Neurol. **16**(8), 661–676 (2017)
7. Gibson, E., et al.: NiftyNet: a deep-learning platform for medical imaging. Comput. Meth. Prog. Biomed. **158**, 113–122 (2018)
8. Helms, G., et al.: Increased SNR and reduced distortions by averaging multiple gradient echo signals in 3D flash imaging of the human brain at 3T. J. Magn. Reson. Imaging Official J. Int. Soc. Magn. Reson. Med. **29**(1), 198–204 (2009)
9. Jog, A., et al.: MR image synthesis by contrast learning on neighborhood ensembles. Med. Image Anal. **24**(1), 63–76 (2015)
10. Jog, A., Fischl, B.: Pulse sequence resilient fast brain segmentation. In: Frangi, A.F., Schnabel, J.A., Davatzikos, C., Alberola-López, C., Fichtinger, G. (eds.) MICCAI 2018. LNCS, vol. 11072, pp. 654–662. Springer, Cham (2018). https://doi.org/10.1007/978-3-030-00931-1_75
11. Milletari, F., et al.: V-net: Fully convolutional neural networks for volumetric medical image segmentation. In: In 2016 Fourth International Conference on 3D Vision, pp. 565–571. IEEE (2016)
12. Rooney, W.D., et al.: Magnetic field and tissue dependencies of human brain longitudinal 1h2o relaxation in vivo. Magn. Reson. Med. Official J. Int. Soc. Magn. Reson. Med. **57**(2), 308–318 (2007)
13. Shinohara, R.T., et al.: Volumetric analysis from a harmonized multisite brain MRI study of a single subject with multiple sclerosis. Am. J. Neuroradiol. **38**(8), 1501–1509 (2017)
14. Wang, J., et al.: Optimizing the magnetization-prepared rapid gradient-echo (mprage) sequence. PloS one **9**(5), e96899 (2014)
15. Weiskopf, N., et al.: Quantitative multi-parameter mapping of r1, pd*, mt, and r2* at 3t: a multi-center validation. Front. Neurosci. **7**, 95 (2013)

3D Medical Image Synthesis
by Factorised Representation
and Deformable Model Learning

Thomas Joyce$^{(\boxtimes)}$ and Sebastian Kozerke

ETH Zurich, Zürich, Switzerland
joycet@ethz.ch

Abstract. In this paper we propose a model for controllable synthesis of 3D (volumetric) medical image data. The model is comprised of three components which are learnt simultaneously from unlabelled data through self-supervision: (i) a multi-tissue anatomical model, (ii) a probability distribution over deformations of this anatomical model, and, (iii) a probability distribution over 'renderings' of the anatomical model (where a rendering defines the relationship between anatomy and resulting pixel intensities). After training, synthetic data can be generated by sampling the deformation and rendering distributions. To encourage meaningful correspondence in the learnt anatomical model the renderer is kept simple during training, however once trained the (deformed) anatomical model provides *dense* multi-class segmentation masks for all training volumes, which can be used directly for state-of-the-art conditional image synthesis. This factored model based approach to data synthesis has a number of advantages: Firstly, it allows for coherent synthesis of realistic 3D data, as it is only necessary to learn low dimensional generative models (over deformations and renderings) rather than over the high dimensional 3D images themselves. Secondly, as a by-product of the anatomical model we implicitly learn a dense correspondence between all training volumes, which can be used for registration, or one-shot segmentation (through label transfer). Lastly, the factored representation allows for modality transfer (rendering one image in the modality of another), and meaningful interpolation between volumes. We demonstrate the proposed approach on cardiac MR, and multi-modal abdominal MR/CT datasets.

Keywords: 3D image synthesis · Conditional image generation · Cardiac magnetic resonance · Anatomical model · Generative model

1 Introduction

Image synthesis techniques have improved significantly over the last few years, and synthetic data has been effectively leveraged in a broad range of medical imaging tasks [2], including segmentation [3], classification [4] and reconstruction [5]. However, despite these results current medical image synthesis

© Springer Nature Switzerland AG 2019
N. Burgos et al. (Eds.): SASHIMI 2019, LNCS 11827, pp. 110–119, 2019.
https://doi.org/10.1007/978-3-030-32778-1_12

approaches have a number of limitations that prevent them from being applied even more widely. Firstly, although there are now many papers demonstrating impressive high resolution results of 2D image generation [6], there is still limited progress on the generation of 3D (volumetric) images. Secondly, controllable image synthesis, in which image generation can be meaningfully conditioned on some input (such as a dense semantic mask) is under explored in the medical setting. Lastly, synthesis of labelled data (e.g. data with multi-class segmentation masks) is strictly more useful than unlabelled image synthesis, but many papers focus on unlabelled image synthesis, or synthesis restricted to binary classes [2,4]

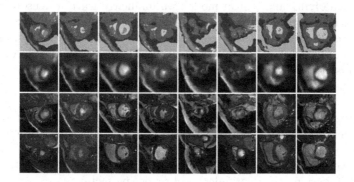

Fig. 1. Example synthetic cardiac MR images from the proposed model. The first row shows random samples from the learnt multi-tissue anatomical model, the second and third rows show synthetic images generated conditioned on those anatomical model samples with the simple and SPADE-based [1] renderers respectively. The final row shows the closest (l_2-norm) real image in the (augmented) training set. (Note that the model synthesises 3D volumes and we visualise random slices).

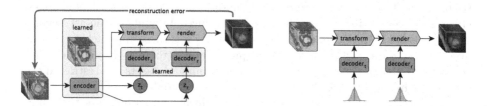

Fig. 2. An overview of the proposed approach. During training (left) the anatomical model, encoder and decoder networks are learnt through self-supervision. Image volumes are encoded to latent vectors z_t (encoding the transformation) and z_r (encoding the rendering), which are both encouraged to have a Gaussian distribution. When synthesising data (right) Gaussian noise is fed to the decoders, and a syhtnetic volume is produced by realistically deforming and rendering the learnt anatomical model.

In this paper we propose an approach to address these problems. We introduce a model for data synthesis that learns a factored representation of 3D medical data which it then leverages to generate diverse and realistic synthetic images with corresponding dense labels (Fig. 1). Specifically, the model learns an *anatomical* factor, which captures the spatial structure of the data, and a *rendering* factor, which describes how the anatomy is rendered to a final image. The anatomical factor is represented as a deformation of a single multi-tissue anatomical model. This anatomical model is also learnt during training. The rendering factor then describes how the various tissues translate into final pixel intensities (see Fig. 2).

We demonstrate that this explicitly enforced factorisation enables the model to synthesise realistic 3D data. Moreover, the proposed framework also provides additional benefits. As all data are represented by (different deformations of) the same underlying anatomical model, we implicitly learn a dense correspondence between all training volumes, as well as between all synthesised images. We demonstrate that this dense correspondence facilitates few-shot, and even one-shot, segmentation via label propagation. Moreover, this dense correspondence allows us to co-register volumes, or to directly apply random realistic deformations.

After training, the anatomical model provides a dense semantic segmentation for every volume in the training set. As a second step we demonstrate that such dense segmentation masks can be used with state-of-the-art conditional image synthesis models [1] to generate sharp, high resolution synthetic image data, and that moreover, this synthesis is controllable in a natural and readily interpretable way, through varying the anatomical and rendering factors.

2   Related Work

Image synthesis has seen impressive recent development [6,7], and provides a powerful approach to enlarging training sets for arbitrary downstream tasks [2,8]. A standard generative model (such as the original GAN [9], or DCGAN [10]) is able to synthesise images *similar to*[1] those in a large set of example images. Given sufficient training data the images produced by state-of-the-art generative models are both realistic and diverse [6]. However, these approaches generate unsegmented data, and there is no (interpretable) control over the specific image generated. Further, the requirement for large training datasets can restrict application in a medical image context, where data is limited.

Various approaches have been developed which help to mitigate these limitations. To address the lack of labels a common approach is to generate labelled data in the target modality from labelled data in another modality through domain transfer [3], however this requires suitable auxiliary labelled data. To achieve controllable image synthesis various conditional generative models have been proposed [2]. Relevant here, a number of recent works have explored controllable synthesis of natural images conditioned on dense segmentation masks [1,11]. These methods have produced exceptional results, but the requirement for dense segmentation masks prohibits straightforward application

---

[1] Broadly, the hope is that the synthetic images are drawn from the same probability distribution over images as the training data was.

to medical images, especially in the 3D case. Alternatively the labels can by synthesised as part of the data (e.g. as additional channels), but this significantly increases the data dimensionality and does not facilitate controllable synthesis.

Lastly, a number of methods that straddle the line between augmentation and synthesis have been proposed, and generate realistic 3D data through shape-model based image deformations [8,12], or from in silico phantoms [13]. However, direct generation of 3D (volumetric) medical image data, to the best of our knowledge, has not yet been demonstrated.

Factored representation learning, i.e. learning representation in which we disentangle "[d]ifferent explanatory factors of the data [that] tend to change independently of each other" [14], is a growing topic in both machine learning and medical image analysis. However, it has recently been shown that factorisation without guiding prior knowledge is not beneficial in general, and the representations learnt do not facilitate improvement in down-stream tasks [15]. In this work our factorisation is explicitly grounded, relying on the fact that medical images result from both a patient's anatomy and an imaging procedure. We make use of this prior knowledge to learn a powerful model without labelled data. Previous work has demonstrated the benefit of factorisation of medical images for segmentation tasks [16,17], and outside of medical imaging there have also been demonstrations of factored representations leveraged to implicitly register data, e.g. on 2D face images [18].

3   Proposed Approach

In this section we describe the proposed approach. A schematic of the connections between the various model components is shown in Fig. 3, and below we describe each element of the model in detail.

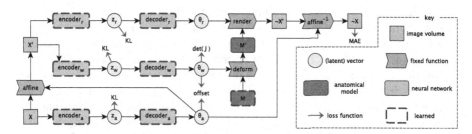

Fig. 3. An overview of the proposed model. An image volume X is given as input, from which the parameters for an affine transform (θ_a) are predicted through a variational encoder-decoder (VED) network (with latent representation z_a). This affine transformation is applied to X producing X'. Next, parameters for a non-linear transformation (deformation) θ_w are predicted from X' (via another VED), and this deformation is applied to the learnt anatomical model M yielding M'. Next, a final VED predicts parameters θ_r from X', and these parameters are used to render M', i.e. map it to an image. Finally the rendered image is aligned with the input X by applying the inverse affine transform. During training the encoder networks, decoder networks, and the anatomical model M are learnt. The other components have no learnable parameters.

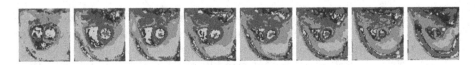

Fig. 4. Example of a $8 \times 64 \times 64 \times 6$ voxel learnt anatomical model. The model was learnt with six tissue types and then clustered into six classes for visualisation with one color per class. The base to apical slices are shown from left to right. It can be seen that, although learnt without supervision, various anatomical parts are clearly visible, such as the ventricular cavities, the myocardium and the chest wall.

Anatomical Model. The proposed approach involves learning an anatomical model M: a multi-channel volume of size $S \times W \times H \times C$. S is the number of slices in the volume, W and H are the in-plane image dimensions (in pixels), and C is the number of channels. C can be seen as a hyper-parameter which defines the maximum number of different 'materials' (or 'tissue types') in the anatomical model. We restrict M such that for every voxel the values across the channels dimension sum to one. Intuitively, this can be understood as letting the values across the channel dimension represent the relative proportion of each tissue type found in each voxel. To implement the model we directly learn the (unconstrained) values of a volume M_{pre} (identical in size to M) during training, and define $M := softmax(M_{pre})$ where the softmax is over the channel dimension. An example of a learnt anatomical model is shown in Fig. 4.

Variational Encoder-Decoder Networks. Our model employs three variational encoder-decoder [19] networks (VEDs). Each of these networks consists of an encoder, which encodes the input to a latent vector, and a decoder, which maps this latent vector to the required output. The first VED takes as input the original image volume X and predicts affine transformation parameters θ_a. The second VED takes as input the affine-transformed image volume X' and predicts the non-linear warp parameters θ_w, and the third VED also takes as input the affine-transformed input volume X', and predicts the rendering parameters θ_r. We define $\theta_t = \{\theta_a, \theta_w\}$, i.e. the parameters of the full transformation. We employ the VED approach so that, as in the variational auto-encoder [19], we learn a low-dimensional latent representation for each input, and during training we encourage the posterior over the latent space to be a standard Gaussian distribution, allowing us to use the model in a generative way by sampling z_t and z_r for standard Gaussian distributions (see Fig. 2). Each encoder is three 32 channel $3 \times 3 \times 3$ convolutions with stride $(1, 2, 2)$ then two 128 neuron dense layers and a final dense layer of the required size with no activation. The decoders are the same as the dense layers of the encoders. We use ReLU activations throughout. The latent spaces z_w, z_a, z_r are size 64, 16, 16.

Transforms. The first step of the pipeline is to transform the input volume using an affine transform such that the input is approximately aligned with the anatomical model. After this transformation the model and input volume have the same overall orientation and scale, but are not co-registered at the individual voxel level as this requires a further non-linear registration step (see below). The affine transform is specified by $\theta_a \in \mathbb{R}^{12}$. Note that later in the processing we invert the predicted affine transform. This is only possible if the matrix is non-singular, however we found that the reconstruction cost itself is sufficient to ensure this condition is met, and no additional regularisation is required.

The next step is to perform a non-linear deformation of the anatomical model M to produce a dense correspondence with the (affine-aligned) input volume X'. We investigated several deformation methods but found that directly predicting a dense offset field (with suitable regularisation, see Sect. 3 for details), produced the best results. Thus $\theta_w \in \mathbb{R}^{S \times W \times H \times 3}$. Although this deformation is not required to be invertible by the model, encouraging invertibility provides strong regularisation, and allows for co-registration of volumes via their predicted deformations.

Rendering. The final step is to convert the warped anatomical model into an image. We refer to this step as 'rendering'. In order to encourage the anatomical model to capture as much information as possible we restrict the renderer to a simple network that assigns a single colour per tissue. Specifically, the simple render learns just C weights (and a bias) and performs a weighted sum of the anatomical model's channels to yield the final image. After training the model we then learn a 2D SPADE-based renderer [1], leveraging the predicted dense segmentation masks, which we up-sample to 128×128.

Loss Function. We train the model end-to-end to minimise the mean-absolute-error of the reconstruction, L_{MAE}. Additionally, we minimise the KL divergences of z_t and z_r from standard Gaussian distributions (loss component L_{KL}). This is done using the reparameterisation trick, as in the original VAE [19].

To regularise the non-linear transformation (and encourage invertability) we minimise $L_{det(J)} = |1 - det(J)|$, where $det(J)$ is the determinant of the Jacoboian of the non-linear transformation. We also minimise the overall offset resulting from the combination of the affine and non-linear transformations, L_{offset}, this encourages the model to minimise the distance between a voxel's initial position in the model and its final position after both transformations. We weight the z direction of this offset to account for the volume's non-isotropic resolution.

The overall loss function is defined as $\lambda_1 L_{MAE} + \lambda_2 L_{KL} + \lambda_3 L_{det(J)} + \lambda_4 L_{offset}$ where λs are hyper-parameters that appropriately scale each loss and determine their relative importances, set empirically to 1, 0.001, 0.1 and 0.0001 respectively.

4   Experiment Details

4.1   Data and Pre-processing

We make use of two datasets: **ACDC** (Automated Cardiac Diagnosis Challenge) [20] consists of cardiac magnetic resonance images (MRI) of 100 patients, both healthy (20%) and unhealthy (80%). We preprocess the data by resampling to 1.3×1.3 mm in-plane resolution (keeping the inter-slice resolution unchanged). We then crop the in-plane image to a 144 × 144 pixels. In total we have 200 (100 end-systolic (ES) and 100 end-diastolic (ED)) volumes, each with an average of 9 slices. The **CHAOS** (Combined Healthy Abdominal Organ Segmentation) dataset [21–23] consists of Abdominal CT and MRI images from different patients. Here we use the CT data and the T1-DUAL in phase MR images, and preprocess the data as done for ACDC, additionally downsampling to 8 slices.

4.2   Training Details

In all experiments we first train the proposed model for 2,000 epochs using Adam [24] with default parameters, a learning rate of 0.01, and a batch size of 32. We use online data augmentation to enhance the seen data variation: we randomly select an 8 × 128 × 128 sub-volume, down-sample to 8 × 64 × 64.

After training the initial model we then train the SPADE-based renderer on 2D image-mask pairs (at 128 × 128 resolution). The voxels in the anatomical model are not discrete classes, but rather contain ratios of the tissues. Thus, in order to make discrete multi-class segmentation maps we perform K-means clustering on the voxels. This produces K distinct classes of voxel, which we use for the segmentation map. We then train the original SPADE model on our data.

5   Results

2D and 3D Synthesis. Given Gaussian noise as input, the learnt model synthesises coherent 3D volumes (from which a 2D slice can then be randomly sampled if required, see Fig. 1). We visualise two example volumes in Fig. 5. As can be seen, the data is anatomically coherent both within and between slices, and the synthetic data is not simply memorised from the training set.

Label Transfer. We evaluate few-shot segmentation on ACDC by using a small number of volumes to learn labels for the anatomical model, then encoding test volumes and evaluating the Dice between the real labels and the labels of the warped anatomical model. Averaged over 10 splits we achieve Dice scores of 69%, 67%, 63%, 60% and 55% for 150, 50, 10, 3 and 1 shot label transfer respectively (over three classes: myocardium and both ventricular blood-pools). Although these results are lower than those produced with supervision they are on par with results learned from unpaired data [25]. It should also be noted that the training data is used only to learn the labels for the anatomical model, the model itself remains constant, and thus the model's correspondence is at least 69%.

Latent Space Interpolation. First we perform Pseudo 4D synthesis. We take the ES and ED volumes from an ACDC patient and interpolate (in the latent space) between their anatomical model deformations. This produces a smooth

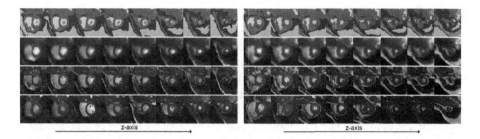

Fig. 5. Two example 3D synthetic image sets ($128 \times 128 \times 8$ voxels). Each 3D image consist of 8 short-axis slices. The first three rows show the sampled anatomical model, result of the simple renderer, and result of the SPADE-based renderer. The final row shows, for each generated slice, the most similar slice (l_2 norm) from the (augmented) training set.

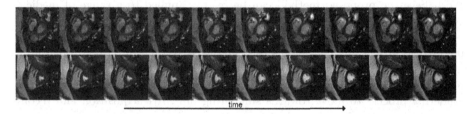

Fig. 6. Example "4D" synthesis ($8 \times 128 \times 128$ voxels, 10 frames). Each frame consist of 8 short-axis slices, here we show two slices due to space constraints. See text for details.

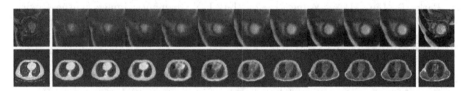

Fig. 7. Latent interpolation on ACDC (top) and CHAOS (bottom). In each row the left and right most images are real, and the ten central images show reconstructions (using the simple renderer) when interpolating linearly between the latent representations of the outer images. It can be seen that both the shape and intensities smoothly transition. Note the second row shows a multi-modal transition between CT and MR.

continuum of anatomies between the two cardiac phases. We then render all volumes using the SPADE-based renderer, resulting in 4D data for half of a cardiac cycle. The results are shown in Fig. 6. As only ES and ED frames were used for training the figure should be taken more as an example of the models ability to meaningfully interpolate, rather then as realistic synthesis of cardiac motion, as the intricacies of the cardiac dynamics may not be captured. We further examine the learnt latent space of the model through additional interpolations in Fig. 7. In particular, results on CHAOS demonstrate multi-modal interpolation.

6 Conclusion and Discussion

We have presented a method for synthesis of medical image data via a learnt anatomical model and factored representation. Image volumes are represented as an anatomical factor z_t (model deformation) and an rendering factor z_r. Factoring the task in this way breaks the synthesis process into two simpler problems which can be solved in parallel. Further, the approach has a number of benefits: it emulates the real factored nature of medical image generation into patient and protocol, learns a multi-tissue (generative) shape model, implicitly co-registers all volumes (i.e. both training and synthesised), and allows for multi-modal learning by explicitly capturing the shared anatomical and discrepant appearance information. Additionally, it yields dense segmentation masks for all volumes, and this combined with the model's modular nature means the render can be replaced by a state-of-the-art conditional synthesis model after training. We believe the proposed method can be readily applied to a range of medical synthesis tasks.

Lastly, our method uses a voxelised anatomical model. Future work looking instead at learning continuous (e.g. mesh-based) anatomy would open up a number of research directions, e.g. allowing simulating k-space acquisition and reconstruction without committing "inverse crime" [26]. This would allow the rendering process to move towards simulating full MRI acquisition and reconstruction.

References

1. Park, T., Liu, M.-Y., Wang, T.-C., Zhu, J.-Y.: Semantic image synthesis with spatially-adaptive normalization. In: Proceedings of the IEEE Conference on Computer Vision and Pattern Recognition (2019)
2. Yi, X., Walia, E., Babyn, P.: Generative adversarial network in medical imaging: a review. arXiv preprint arXiv:1809.07294 (2018)
3. Chartsias, A., Joyce, T., Dharmakumar, R., Tsaftaris, S.A.: Adversarial image synthesis for unpaired multi-modal cardiac data. In: Tsaftaris, S.A., Gooya, A., Frangi, A.F., Prince, J.L. (eds.) SASHIMI 2017. LNCS, vol. 10557, pp. 3–13. Springer, Cham (2017). https://doi.org/10.1007/978-3-319-68127-6_1
4. Frid-Adar, M., Diamant, I., Klang, E., Amitai, M., Goldberger, J., Greenspan, H.: Gan-based synthetic medical image augmentation for increased CNN performance in liver lesion classification. Neurocomputing **321**, 321–331 (2018)
5. Quan, T.M., Nguyen-Duc, T., Jeong, W.-K.: Compressed sensing MRI reconstruction using a generative adversarial network with a cyclic loss. IEEE Trans. Med. Imaging **37**(6), 1488–1497 (2018)
6. Brock, A., Donahue, J., Simonyan, K.: Large scale GAN training for high fidelity natural image synthesis. arXiv preprint arXiv:1809.11096 (2018)
7. Razavi, A., van den Oord, A., Vinyals, O.: Generating diverse high-fidelity images with VQ-VAE-2. arXiv preprint arXiv:1906.00446 (2019)
8. Corral Acero, J., et al.: SMOD - data augmentation based on statistical models of deformation to enhance segmentation in 2D cine cardiac MRI. In: Coudière, Y., Ozenne, V., Vigmond, E., Zemzemi, N. (eds.) FIMH 2019. LNCS, vol. 11504, pp. 361–369. Springer, Cham (2019). https://doi.org/10.1007/978-3-030-21949-9_39

9. Goodfellow, I.: Generative adversarial nets. In: Advances in neural information processing systems, pp. 2672–2680 (2014)
10. Radford, A., Metz, L., Chintala, S.: Unsupervised representation learning with deep convolutional generative adversarial networks. arXiv (2015)
11. Wang, T.-C., Liu, M.-Y., Zhu, J.-Y., Tao, A., Kautz, J., Catanzaro, B.: High-resolution image synthesis and semantic manipulation with conditional GANs. In: Proceedings of the IEEE CVPR, pp. 8798–8807 (2018)
12. Bansal, A., Sheikh, Y., Ramanan, D.: Shapes and context: in-the-wild image synthesis & manipulation. arXiv preprint arXiv:1906.04728 (2019)
13. Wissmann, L., Santelli, C., Segars, W.P., Kozerke, S.: MRXCAT: realistic numerical phantoms for cardiovascular magnetic resonance. J. Cardiovasc. Magn. Reson. $16(1)$, 63 (2014)
14. Bengio, Y., Courville, A., Vincent, P.: Representation learning: a review and new perspectives. IEEE TPAMI $35(8)$, 1798–1828 (2013)
15. Locatello, F., Bauer, S., Lucic, M., Gelly, S., Schölkopf, B., Bachem, O.: Challenging common assumptions in the unsupervised learning of disentangled representations. arXiv preprint arXiv:1811.12359 (2018)
16. Chartsias, A., et al.: Factorised representation learning in cardiac image analysis. arXiv:1903.09467 (2019)
17. Xia, T., Chartsias, A., Tsaftaris, S.A.: Adversarial pseudo healthy synthesis needs pathology factorization. arXiv preprint arXiv:1901.07295 (2019)
18. Shu, Z., Sahasrabudhe, M., Alp Güler, R., Samaras, D., Paragios, N., Kokkinos, I.: Deforming autoencoders: unsupervised disentangling of shape and appearance. In: Ferrari, V., Hebert, M., Sminchisescu, C., Weiss, Y. (eds.) ECCV 2018. LNCS, vol. 11214, pp. 664–680. Springer, Cham (2018). https://doi.org/10.1007/978-3-030-01249-6_40
19. Kingma, D.P., Welling, M.: Auto-encoding variational Bayes. arXiv preprint arXiv:1312.6114 (2013)
20. Bernard, O., et al.: Deep learning techniques for automatic MRI cardiac multi-structures segmentation and diagnosis: is the problem solved? IEEE Trans. Med. Imaging $37(11)$, 2514–2525 (2018)
21. Selver, M.A.: Exploring brushlet based 3D textures in transfer function specification for direct volume rendering of abdominal organs. IEEE Trans. Vis. Comput. Graph. $21(2)$, 174–187 (2014)
22. Selvi, E., Selver, M.A., Kavur, A.E., Guzelis, C., Dicle, O.: Segmentation of abdominal organs from MR images using multi-level hierarchical classification. J. Fac. Eng. Arch. Gazi Univ. $30(3)$, 533–546 (2015)
23. Selver, M.A.: Segmentation of abdominal organs from CT using a multi-level, hierarchical neural network strategy. Comput. Methods Programs Biomed. $113(3)$, 830–852 (2014)
24. Kingma, D.P., Ba, J.: Adam: a method for stochastic optimization. arXiv preprint arXiv:1412.6980 (2014)
25. Joyce, T., Chartsias, A., Tsaftaris, S.A.: Deep multi-class segmentation without ground-truth labels (2018)
26. Wirgin, A.: The inverse crime. arXiv preprint math-ph/0401050 (2004)

Cycle-Consistent Training for Reducing Negative Jacobian Determinant in Deep Registration Networks

Dongyang Kuang[1,2]( )

[1] University of Ottawa, Ottawa, Canada
dykuang@outlook.com
[2] University of Texas – Austin, Austin, Texas, USA

Abstract. Image registration is a fundamental step in medical image analysis. Ideally, the transformation that registers one image to another should be a diffeomorphism that is both invertible and smooth. Traditional methods like geodesic shooting study the problem via differential geometry, with theoretical guarantees that the resulting transformation will be smooth and invertible. Most previous research using unsupervised deep neural networks for registration address the smoothness issue directly either by using a local smoothness constraint (typically, a spatial variation loss), or by designing network architectures enhancing spatial smoothness. In this paper, we examine this problem from a different angle by investigating possible training mechanisms/tasks that will help the network avoid predicting transformations with negative Jacobians and produce smoother deformations. The proposed cycle consistent idea reduces the number of folding locations in predicted deformations without making changes to the hyperparameters or the architecture used in the existing backbone registration network. Code for the paper is available at https://github.com/dykuang/Medical-image-registration.

Keywords: Unsupervised registration · Cycle consistent training · Folding deduction

1 Introduction

Image registration is a key element of medical image analysis. Most state-of-the-art registration algorithms, such as ANTs [1], can utilize geometric methods that are guaranteed to produce smooth invertible deformations that are much desired in medical image registrations. A revolution is taking place in the last couple of years in the application of machine learning methods. Especially, the method of convolutional neural networks have made impressive progresses and caused a lot of attentions. While recent registration networks can make predictions of the nonlinear transformation much faster and obtain registration accuracy comparable to or better than traditional methods, they usually do not have theoretical guarantees on the smoothness or invertibility of their predicted deformations.

© Springer Nature Switzerland AG 2019
N. Burgos et al. (Eds.): SASHIMI 2019, LNCS 11827, pp. 120–129, 2019.
https://doi.org/10.1007/978-3-030-32778-1_13

Supervised methods, such as in [8, 11, 13], learn from known reference deformations for training data – either actual "ground truth" in the case of synthetic image pairs, or deformations computed by other automatic or semi-automatic methods. They usually do not have problems of smoothness, but still rely on other tools such as ANTs running ahead to produce desired transformations. The registration problem is much harder in the setting of unsupervised methods. Most of the early unsupervised approaches like [2, 7, 10, 12, 14] take the idea of spatial transformer (ST) [4]. This spatial transformer used in registration usually consists of two basic functional units: a deformation unit and a sampling unit. With input x (source image) and y (target image) stacked as an ordered pair, the deformation unit produces a static displacement field $\mathbf{u} : \mathcal{R}^3 \rightarrow \mathcal{R}^3$. The warped image $\tilde{y}$ is then constructed in the sampling unit by interpolating the source image with $\mathbf{u}$ via $\tilde{y} = x(Id + \mathbf{u})$, where Id is the identity map. As a summary, the right action of diffeomorphism ϕ on image x is approximated by $\phi \cdot x = x \circ \phi^{-1} \approx x(Id + \mathbf{u})$. The smoothness constraint on $\mathbf{u}$ is usually addressed by regularizing its derivative $D\mathbf{u}$. The work [2] is one representative and Fig. 1 shows the work flow of the idea introduced as above. The whole network is trained so that it minimizes the loss: $CC(y, \tilde{y}) + \lambda \|D\mathbf{u}\|_{l_2}$, where CC stands for cross correlation loss and λ is a hyperparameter controlling the strength of the regularization.

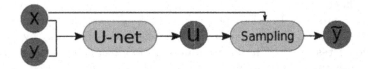

Fig. 1. An overview of the registration network usually used for registration. The popular U-net architecture [9] is used as the deformation unit for generating the displacement field.

These work emphasize more on the accuracy and efficiency of registration when compared to classical methods but usually did not put equal attentions on checking geometric properties such as smoothness, invertibility or orientation preservation for the predicted deformations. Particularly, Jacobian determinant of the predicted transformations i.e. $\det(D\phi^{-1}) \approx \det(Id + D\mathbf{u})$ from a neural network can very likely be negative at multiple locations. This "folding" issue during prediction may still persist even when one increases regularization strength of $D\mathbf{u}$ (see Fig. 2). Additionally, the value of this hyper-parameter is usually difficult to set in practice in order to reach a good balance between nice geometrical properties[1] and registration accuracy, since larger λ values often cause smaller deformations reducing the accuracy.

---

[1] In the paper, it will mainly refer to smoothness, invertibility and particularly, transformations has positive Jacobian determinant everywhere.

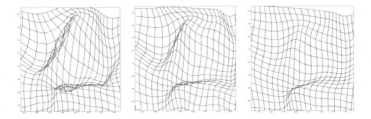

Fig. 2. A snapshot of at the same location of the projected warped grid with different regularization strength. From left to right, the network is trained with $\lambda = 1, 2, 4$ separately. The same location is also used in Fig. 7.

Built upon previous research, state-of-the-art works like [3] proposes a probabilistic VoxelMorph (Prob-VM) design that takes a reparametrization trick and inserts an "integration layer" trying to produce smoother deformation. From modeling point of view, this process-oriented modeling is usually difficult and requires much effort to design a new architecture ahead of time that is proved to be effective later on general data. In order to make an easier modeling process avoiding going inside the box to handcraft an ideal architecture, one can keep the original network with possible flaws untouched but instead seek a different training mechanism/task that is possible to achieve better regularization implicitly. This thought of task-oriented modeling may reveal an alternative way for solving the same problem. In this paper, we take this direction and propose a cycle consistent design for training unsupervised registration networks by assigning an additional task to it. The idea requires no modifications of backbone network's architectures, form of loss functions or hyperparameters used, hence can be used upon any well-known backbone registration networks. From our experiments with VoxelMorph as the backbone network, the proposed idea reduces chances of negative Jacobian determinant in its predicted transformations and can achieve comparable results with Prob-VM.

2   Related Work

To author's best knowledge when completing this paper, [15] and [3] are most relevant research in reducing negative Jacobian. Our proposed idea represents a different strategy in solving the problem (see Fig. 3). [15] designed an inverse consistent network and argued adding an explicit "anti-folding constraint" to prevent folding in predicted transformation. Different from his work, we do not create new forms of losses targeting on specific properties, but focuses on discovering possible training mechanisms/tasks that will help better regularize the network in a general way. [3] is developed upon [2] by integrating an variational auto-encoder design and inserting an integration layer that "integrates" initial velocity field to get the final displacements. Unlike their work on modifying backbone architectures for better performance, the cycle consistent idea in this paper leaves the backbone network untouched but achieves regularization implicitly by adding one more task of recovering the source image from its already predicted image during training. This additional task is meant to help narrow the solution domain where non-smooth or non-invertible transformations are hardly inside during optimization.

3 Proposed Methods

3.1 Cycle Consistent Design

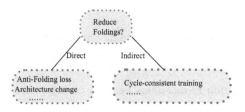

Fig. 3. Two directions for addressing folding issues in prediction.

From the mathematical point of view, the transformations used in registration tasks should ideally be diffeomorphisms so that topological properties are not changed during the transformations. In order to approximate the ideal deformation, training of the network should also respect this invertibility property. In fields such as computer vision, there have already been research such as [16] utilizing this idea for better quality control of cross-domain image generations. In their work, they defined two joint cycle consistent loops for better training two separate generative adversarial networks for unpaired image-to-image translation back-and-forth. We use a related idea in a different setting here for regularizing the predicted static displacement field. This "cycle consistent" idea does not involve new form of losses but forces the same network to perform a backward prediction trying to recover the input right after it completes the forward prediction. As seen in Fig. 4, the spatial transformer will first predict a warped image $\tilde{y}$ and the corresponding displacement field $\mathbf{u}_{x\to\tilde{y}}$ with the stacked source image x and target image y. This predicted warped image $\tilde{y}$ (now as source) is then stacked with the original source image x (now as target). They will be fed into the same spatial transformer to produce a reconstruction $\tilde{x}$ for x and corresponding inverted displacement field $\mathbf{u}_{\tilde{y}\to\tilde{x}}$. The whole network is trained with the cycle consistent loss:

$$CC(y, \tilde{y}) + \lambda||D\mathbf{u}_{x\to\tilde{y}}||_{l_2} + CC(x, \tilde{x}) + \lambda||D\mathbf{u}_{\tilde{y}\to\tilde{x}}||_{l_2} \qquad (1)$$

While it is straightforward that this design directly addresses the invertibility of the network, the cycle constraint task also contributes to the task of learning a smooth solution in an indirect way: the design regularizes the network by forcing the spatial transformer to learn a solution and its possible inverse at the same time. This helps the network rule out transformations that are not cycle consistent during optimization. This design also does not add any additional learnable parameters to the original spatial transformer and can be trained as equally efficient.

Though similar, this idea is also different from bi-directional registrations where the target image will also be warped towards the source image during optimization. In our design, the target image will never be warped. To be more specific, given loss function L and input source-target image pair (x, y), the neural network with parameters θ learns the mapping f to transform x towards y:

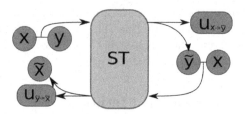

Fig. 4. A diagram illustrating the cycle consistent design.

$y \approx f(\theta; (x, y))$. The two optimization problems can be vaguely summarized as below in Table 1:

Table 1. Different object function optimization formulations between bi-directional registration and cycle-consistent training.

Methods	Formulations of optimization
Bi-direction:	$\arg\min_\theta L(y, f(\theta; x, y)) + L(x, f(\theta; y, x))$
Cycle-consistent:	$\arg\min_\theta L(y, f(\theta; x, y)) + L(x, f(\theta; f(\theta; x, y), x))$

Bi-direction registration uses both pairs (x, y) and (y, x) as inputs, while the cycle-consistent training only uses (x, y). They are equivalent if there exists a "perfect" deformation that aligns the registration pair and this transformation f can be learned with parameters θ during training: $y = f(\theta; (x, y))$.

4   Experiment

4.1   Dataset

We used MindBoggle101 dataset [6] for experiments. Details of data collection and processing, including atlas creation, are described in [6]. In the present paper, we used brain volumes consisting of the following three named subsets of Mindboggle101:

- NKI-RS-22: "Nathan Kline Institute/Rockland sample"
- NKI-TRT-20: "Nathan Kline Institute/Test–Retest"
- OASIS-TRT-20: "Open Access Series of Imaging Studies/ Test–Retest".

Each image has a dimension of $182 \times 218 \times 182$, we truncated the margin reducing the size to $144 \times 180 \times 144$. These images are already linearly aligned to MNI152 space. We also normalized the intensity of each brain volume to $[0, 1]$ by its maximum voxel intensity. Figure 5 shows one subject of the dataset with two annotated labels. Labels used in Mindboggle101 data set are cortex surface labels. Their geometrical complexity leads to more challenging registration tasks, especially for neural network approaches. In the following experiments, the original VoxelMorph network [2] will be used as the backbone network. This backbone network alone, it with cycle consistent design and the probabilistic VoxelMorph will be compared. The backbone method and the method with cycle consistent design are trained with $\lambda = 1$. Unless specifically stated, epochs $= 10$ and "Adam" optimizer [5] with learning rate 10^{-4} are used for all the three networks.

We access the accuracy of predicted registration via dice score between ROI labels/masks. For image pair (x, y), each indexed label L_x^i associated with x will be warped with the deformation ϕ predicted from the registration network, dice score is then calculated. A higher dice score usually indicates a better registration.

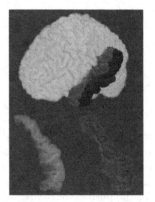

$$Dice(\,(\phi \cdot L_x^i), L_y^i\,) = \frac{2|(\phi \cdot L_x^i) \cap L_y^i|}{|\phi \cdot L_x^i| + |L_y^i|} \qquad (2)$$

We first visualize this metric on test set (OASIS-TRT-20) in Fig. 6. It gives a detailed summary of dice scores on separate regions for registration. All the three neural network approaches appear to provide similar dice scores for most regions and slightly outperform the non-neural-network-based method such as Ants' SyNQuick algorithm. As will be illus-

Fig. 5. One sample with two ROI labels shown. Bottom: the two labels viewed from a different angle

trated later in details, these similar dice scores are actually results of deformations that have different Jacobian properties. The foldings of the deformation is accessed via examining locations where negative Jacobian determinants happen. Let $\mathcal{P}$ be defined as the percentage of voxel locations where the Jacobian determinant is negative over all voxels V, i.e.

$$\mathcal{P} := \frac{\sum \delta(det(D\phi^{-1}) < 0)}{V}.$$

The ideal transformation predicted should have this number as small as possible. To better access the general performance of our proposed methods, we perform a 3-fold validation[2] with the 3 datasets at hand. We summarize this number from different methods into Table 2 for comparison. The author reminds readers that Table 2 is not for the purpose of competing with Prob-VoxelMorph or Ants' SyN-Quick, but simply a demonstration that an indirect task oriented method such as the proposed cycle-consistent training can also achieve comparable registration quality with state-of-the-art method such as Prob-VoxelMorph. To support this, results from some statistical hypothesis tests are organized in Table 3.

---

[2] Each fold will use 2 of the 3 datasets for forming training set and test on the third. Figures 6 and 7 are from the fold when pairs from OAISIS dataset are used as test. This experiment has 1722 training pairs and 380 test pairs.

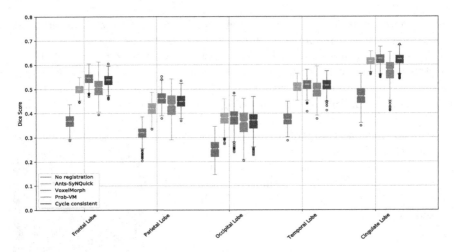

Fig. 6. Mean dice scores of different methods on selected regions. Each point is the mean dice score averaged over corresponding ROI labels per registration pair instead of over the union of labels in that region. Results from SyNQuick algorithm in the ANTs package are also listed as an example for better interpreting these dice scores, but not for the purpose of comparison.

It is clear that Table 2 suggests there are differences of the underlying transformation in terms of the measures introduced as above. From the cross validation results, the baseline method has a mean value of 1.97% locations where Jacobian determinants are negative. When the cycle consistent design is applied, this value drops to 0.13%. In other words, more than 90% of the unsatisfactory locations happening in the baseline prediction are eliminated (H_0 can be rejected with p-value $= 0.02$ in test I). This result is very close to the performance of probabilistic VoxelMorph with 0.03% improvement in $\mu(P)$ (whether to adopt or reject H_0 will depend on one's confidence level with p-value $= 0.05$ in test II) and 0.9% "higher" mean dice score (H_0 cannot be rejected with such a large

Table 2. Summary of metrics with the 3-fold validation, mean (μ) and the standard deviation (σ) calculated over the 3 folds are shown. Since Ants' SyNQuick method does not require training set to register a pair of images, folds split is not appropriate for its evaluation. We only record mean values from registering all the pairs in the whole dataset for comparison.

Method	$\mu(\mathcal{P})$	$\sigma(\mathcal{P})$	$\mu(Dice)$	$\sigma(Dice)$
Ants' SyNQuick	≈ 0		47.63%	
VoxelMorph	1.97%	0.59%	49.83%	0.17%
Prob-VoxelMorph	0.16%	0.05%	47.25%	0.19%
Cycle consistent	**0.13%**	**0.04%**	48.10%	0.86%

Table 3. Some hypothesis tests results summarized from the 3-fold experiments. Abbreviations used: CC for "VoxelMorph with Cycle-Consistent training", VM for "VoxelMorph without Cycle-Consistent training" and PVM for the "Prob-VoxelMorph".

Null Hypothesis H_0:	Test performed	p-value
I: $\mu(\mathcal{P})\|_{CC} \geq \mu(\mathcal{P})\|_{VM}$	One tailed paired t-test	0.02
II: $\mu(\mathcal{P})\|_{CC} \geq \mu(\mathcal{P})\|_{PVM}$	One tailed paired t-test	0.05
III: $\mu(Dice)\|_{CC} = \mu(Dice)\|_{PVM}$	Two tailed paired t-test	0.23

p-value in test III of Table 3, hence this improvement is not statistical significant, the two methods are comparable in this measure). As a summary, these results suggest the two different directions (direct ways as Prob-VoxelMorph and indirect approaches as Cycle-Consistent training) have comparable effects in terms of reducing foldings locations while maintaining registration accuracy.

For better visualization, we also put one slice of the Jacobian determinant map and the projected warped grid on the same slice in Fig. 7. The transformation for visualization used in the figure is predicted on the pair formed by subject OASIS-TRT-3 (source) and subject OASIS-TRT-8 (target).

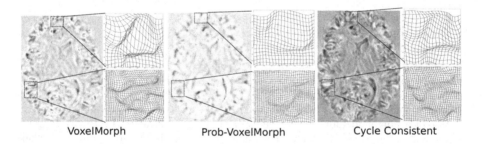

VoxelMorph   Prob-VoxelMorph   Cycle Consistent

Fig. 7. Determinant of Jacobian map and the warped grid projected on the same slice. From left to right: the basline VoxelMorph prediction, the Probabilistic VoxelMorph and baseline with cycle consistent design. Locations where determinants are negative are shown in red. (Color figure online)

Figure 7 shows an example of locations with negative Jacobian determinants. This help give an intuitive view of what happened behind the curtain. From the warped grid columns, one can clearly see networks with cycle consistent design did not change much in locations where the baseline prediction are already smooth but put attentions on foldings and "unfold" them to produce a smoother transformation. Note that the grid shown in the upper right corner of cycle consistent result is smoother compared to the grid shown in the middle of Fig. 2 where the regularization strength is doubled (i.e. $\lambda = 2$). The color map of Prob-VoxelMorph looks pale because there exists at least one location with a large

Jacobian determinant value in this random example. In this case, most locations with Jacobian determinants relatively smaller will be renormalized close to zero during the normalization step when creating the color map.

5 Conclusion

We contribute the idea of cycle-consistent training for reducing locations of negative Jacobian determinants occurred in deformations when a deep neural network is used for unsupervised registration tasks. Unlike most other approaches that address the problem directly by creating new losses or developing new architectures for regularization, this paper focuses on another direction that could bring improvements implicitly by adopting different training mechanisms. The idea does not require changing anything from the backbone network and hence can be used upon arbitrary registration networks. Heuristically, the additional cycle-consistent task during training forces the network to learn recovery transformations at the same time, hence help narrow down the solution domain during optimization. While the theoretical support for this idea still needs to be investigated as part of future research, experiments have shown that this indirect approach is capable of obtaining comparable results with state-of-the-art methods in terms of reducing negative Jacobian determinants while maintaining registration accuracy.

References

1. Avants, B.B., Tustison, N.J., Song, G., Cook, P.A., Klein, A., Gee, J.C.: A reproducible evaluation of ants similarity metric performance in brain image registration. Neuroimage **54**(3), 2033–2044 (2011)
2. Balakrishnan, G., Zhao, A., Sabuncu, M.R., Guttag, J., Dalca, A.V.: An unsupervised learning model for deformable medical image registration. In: Proceedings of the IEEE Conference on Computer Vision and Pattern Recognition, pp. 9252–9260 (2018)
3. Dalca, A.V., Balakrishnan, G., Guttag, J., Sabuncu, M.R.: Unsupervised learning for fast probabilistic diffeomorphic registration. In: Frangi, A.F., Schnabel, J.A., Davatzikos, C., Alberola-López, C., Fichtinger, G. (eds.) MICCAI 2018. LNCS, vol. 11070, pp. 729–738. Springer, Cham (2018). https://doi.org/10.1007/978-3-030-00928-1_82
4. Jaderberg, M., Simonyan, K., Zisserman, A., et al.: Spatial transformer networks. In: Advances in Neural Information Processing Systems, pp. 2017–2025 (2015)
5. Kingma, D.P., Ba, J.: Adam: a method for stochastic optimization. arXiv preprint arXiv:1412.6980 (2014)
6. Klein, A., Tourville, J.: 101 labeled brain images and a consistent human cortical labeling protocol. Front. Neurosci. **6**, 171 (2012)
7. Li, H., Fan, Y.: Non-rigid image registration using fully convolutional networks with deep self-supervision. arXiv preprint arXiv:1709.00799 (2017)

8. Rohé, M.-M., Datar, M., Heimann, T., Sermesant, M., Pennec, X.: SVF-Net: learning deformable image registration using shape matching. In: Descoteaux, M., Maier-Hein, L., Franz, A., Jannin, P., Collins, D.L., Duchesne, S. (eds.) MICCAI 2017. LNCS, vol. 10433, pp. 266–274. Springer, Cham (2017). https://doi.org/10. 1007/978-3-319-66182-7_31
9. Ronneberger, O., Fischer, P., Brox, T.: U-Net: convolutional networks for biomedical image segmentation. In: Navab, N., Hornegger, J., Wells, W.M., Frangi, A.F. (eds.) MICCAI 2015. LNCS, vol. 9351, pp. 234–241. Springer, Cham (2015). https://doi.org/10.1007/978-3-319-24574-4_28
10. Shan, S., et al.: Unsupervised end-to-end learning for deformable medical image registration. arXiv preprint arXiv:1711.08608 (2017)
11. Sokooti, H., de Vos, B., Berendsen, F., Lelieveldt, B.P.F., Išgum, I., Staring, M.: Nonrigid image registration using multi-scale 3D convolutional neural networks. In: Descoteaux, M., Maier-Hein, L., Franz, A., Jannin, P., Collins, D.L., Duchesne, S. (eds.) MICCAI 2017. LNCS, vol. 10433, pp. 232–239. Springer, Cham (2017). https://doi.org/10.1007/978-3-319-66182-7_27
12. Wang, S., Kim, M., Wu, G., Shen, D.: Scalable high performance image registration framework by unsupervised deep feature representations learning. In: Deep Learning for Medical Image Analysis, pp. 245–269. Elsevier (2017)
13. Yang, X., Kwitt, R., Styner, M., Niethammer, M.: Quicksilver: fast predictive image registration-a deep learning approach. NeuroImage **158**, 378–396 (2017)
14. Yoo, I., Hildebrand, D.G.C., Tobin, W.F., Lee, W.-C.A., Jeong, W.-K.: ssEMnet: serial-section electron microscopy image registration using a spatial transformer network with learned features. In: Cardoso, M.J., et al. (eds.) DLMIA/ML-CDS -2017. LNCS, vol. 10553, pp. 249–257. Springer, Cham (2017). https://doi.org/10. 1007/978-3-319-67558-9_29
15. Zhang, J.: Inverse-consistent deep networks for unsupervised deformable image registration. arXiv preprint arXiv:1809.03443 (2018)
16. Zhu, J.Y., Park, T., Isola, P., Efros, A.A.: Unpaired image-to-image translation using cycle-consistent adversarial networks. arXiv preprint (2017)

iSMORE: An Iterative Self Super-Resolution Algorithm

Can Zhao[1]($\boxtimes$), Seoyoung Son[2], Yongsoo Kim[2], and Jerry L. Prince[1]

[1] Department of Electrical and Computer Engineering, Johns Hopkins University, Baltimore, MD, USA
czhao20@jhu.edu
[2] Department of Neural and Behavioral Sciences, Penn State University, Hershey, PA, USA

Abstract. In 3D medical imaging, images with isotropic high resolution (HR) are almost always preferred. In practice, however, many acquired images, including magnetic resonance imaging (MRI) and fluorescence microscopy, have HR in the in-plane directions and low resolution (LR) in the through-plane direction. The blurriness and aliasing artifacts that result cannot be solved by simple interpolation. Instead, many researchers have proposed super-resolution algorithms including state-of-art convolutional neural network (CNN)-based methods that require matched training data that have paired LR/HR examples. Since these data are often unavailable in practice, self super-resolution algorithms that do not need external training data have also been proposed. These self super-resolution methods assume that the in-plane slices are HR, and can therefore be used as HR training data. By degrading them into LR images, 2D CNNs can be trained and then used to restore the images in the through-plane. However, there are two issues with these approaches. The first one is that the assumption of HR in-plane slices is actually not solid since these thick in-plane slices are averaged true HR thin slices. Training on thick slices is equivalent to training on averaged true HR images, which is suboptimal. The second one relates to the 2D CNNs used on 3D volume, which cannot guarantee slice consistency. Regarding both issues as well as the generalizability of algorithm, we made four contributions. We show in this paper that one of the existing 2D CNN-based self super-resolution methods, SMORE, can be further improved by iteratively applying it using 2D or 3D networks, yielding 2D and 3D iSMORE. This iterative framework improves training data from thick slices to thinner slices after each iteration, thus improves super-resolution accuracy after each iteration, and solves the first issue. The second contribution is that it uses a 3D network to preserve slice consistency. The third contribution is the use of an edge-based loss function and noise reduction to enhance the performance. Finally, we perform iSMORE on both MRI and two-photon fluorescence microscopy, which demonstrates its generalizability.

Keywords: Self super-resolution · Deep network · MRI · CNN · Aliasing · Microscopy · SMORE

© Springer Nature Switzerland AG 2019
N. Burgos et al. (Eds.): SASHIMI 2019, LNCS 11827, pp. 130–139, 2019.
https://doi.org/10.1007/978-3-030-32778-1_14

1   Introduction

In 3D medical imaging, high resolution (HR) images with adequate signal-to-noise ratio are always preferred since they provide more anatomical details in clinical and research applications. For magnetic resonance imaging (MRI), such images cost more money, because they require long acquisition times, and are also prone to motion artifacts. For fluorescence microscopy, the resolution is affected by acquisition time, optical settings, and imaging parameters. In practice, a common trade-off is to acquire 3D images with high in-plane resolution and lower through-plane resolution (slice thickness) to save acquisition time.

Degrading through-plane resolution saves time and money and also provides good anatomical detail in the in-plane orientations. However, visualization and analysis in the through-plane direction is difficult or impossible because of the degraded low-resolution (LR). Since most automatic image processing algorithms for 3D analysis require images with isotropic voxels, a common first step is to interpolate the images to meet this requirement. However, interpolation does not restore the missing high-frequency information, which makes the resultant images blurry and (in some cases) rife with aliasing artifacts in the through-plane direction. Consequently, degrading through-plane resolution also degrades the performance of subsequent image processing tasks such as registration and segmentation.

To improve the resolution from such anisotropic acquisitions, researchers have developed many super-resolution algorithms. The state-of-the-art algorithms are CNN-based that require LR/HR paired training data with contrasts and resolutions that closely match the subject data. Unfortunately, such training data is often unavailable. In such cases, self super-resolution (SSR) algorithms that do not require external training data are applicable. Researchers have developed SSR methods that have impressive performance, including Jog et al. [3], Weigert et al. [9] and Zhao et al. [10,11]. These SSR methods assume that the in-plane slices of the subject image are HR and can therefore be used as HR training data. By blurring these images in an in-plane direction, these LR images can be used with the original HR images to train a super-resolution (SR) regressor, which is then applied in the through-plane direction to improve the through-plane resolution of the original data. These methods use different SR regressors. Jog et al. [3] used Anchored Neighborhood Regression [7]; Weigert et al. [9] used a 2D U-net [6]; and Zhao et al. [10,11] used a 2D EDSR network [4], which is one of the state-of-the-art SR networks [8].

Although these SSR algorithms show substantial improvement compared to interpolation, they make an assumption that does not hold up to scrutiny. To explain, consider a thick in-plane slice. Although it has the appearance of HR, it does suffer from through-plane blurring. Edges that pass through the slice orthogonally will appear to be sharp while edges that pass through obliquely will appear to be blurry. An example can be found from the Fig. 2 of Zhao et al. [12]. In this figure, although the axial plane is considered as HR in-plane, we can see that the axial slice of subject image suffered from through-plane blurring, especially near the ventricals. This is because the thick in-plane slices can be considered as averaged HR thin slices, and the averaging brings blurring. Training on thick slices is equivalent to training on averaged true HR images, which is suboptimal. Using these blurred in-plane slices as HR training data will degrade the performance of the SSR algorithm.

Another issue with the previous CNN-based SSR methods is that they all use a 2D CNN on 3D volumes. We know that 2D CNN cannot guarantee slice consistency. This is especially important for 2D protocols, i.e., where images are acquired in 2D and then stacked into 3D volumes. Such 2D acquisitions may not have good slice consistency at the outset, and applying a 2D CNN on them can only make the slice consistency worse. For these 2D protocols, a 3D CNN is preferred, yet this has not been reported for SSR.

The third issue is that the previous SSR methods are only applied in a single image modality with no guidance on how to modify them for other modalities. Weigert et al. [9] developed a method for confocal and light-sheet microscopy data of cells. The SSR method in Jog et al. [3] and one of the SMORE methods, which we refer as SMORE(3D) [10], were developed for MRI acquired from 3D protocols. The other SMORE method, which we refer as SMORE(2D) [10], was developed for MRI acquired from 2D protocols. SMORE has been demonstrated on various of MRI datasets [12], and is therefore chosen as the baseline method. To push it forward, we will demonstrate our methods on two image modalities.

Regarding these issues, this paper describes iSMORE and its four major contributions: (1) an iterative SSR framework, (2) a new 3D CNN for SSR, (3) new loss function and noise reduction, (4) application to two image modalities.

2   Method

2.1   2D iSMORE

A workflow for the iterative framework of iSMORE is shown in Fig. 1(a). Consider an input image $g(x, y, z)$ with anisotropic spatial resolution—i.e, three full-width-half-maxima (FWHM) of the point spread function—of $a \times a \times b$, with $a < b$, and let the HR in-plane directions be x and y and the LR through-plane direction be z. Our goal is to restore a HR image f with the resolution $a \times a \times a$. Traditional SSR methods extract in-plane (xy-plane) slices with resolution $a \times a$ from input image g, which are considered by these methods to be HR data, apply a point spread function (PSF) which mimics the mechanism of LR in the through-plane direction, and simulate LR data with resolution $b \times a$ from these HR data with resolution $a \times a$. The LR/HR pairs are used as training data for super-resolution (SR) networks. The trained SR networks are then applied to LR zx-plane slices with resolution $b \times a$ to restore HR at (ideally) $a \times a$. Finally, the super-resolved zx-plane slices are stacked in y-axis into a 3D volume, which is the SSR result f_1. This traditional SSR procedure is the first iteration in iSMORE.

For input image g, the thick in-plane slices are actually blurred, so they are not perfect training data. On the other hand, the SSR result f_1 has thinner slices. Thus, f_1 has better through-plane resolution than input image g, and serves as better training data than g. Taking in-plane slices from f_1 as HR training data, we subsequently fine-tune the SR network. The fine-tuned network is then applied to input g as in the first iteration, and the SSR result f_2. We iteratively perform these steps until the stop condition is met.

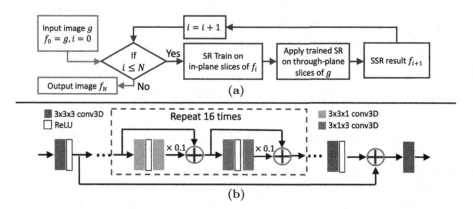

Fig. 1. (a) The framework of iSMORE. The sequence of super-resolution networks (SR) are trained on the SSR result from the previous iteration, and SR is always applied to the input data. (b) Architecture of 3D EDSR

We use SMORE as our baseline SSR method and apply our 2D iterative framework to the SMORE result, yielding 2D iSMORE. Data augmentation for training includes flipping and rotation except for rotation of 90°, which is only used for validation to avoid overfitting.

2.2 3D iSMORE and a New 3D Network

It is problematic to directly train a 3D network to perform SSR. If we degrade the input image g into an LR image with resolution $b \times a \times b$, and train a 3D network to learn the mapping from it to g, then it is wrong to apply the network to the rotated input image g with resolution $b \times a \times a$ because this resolution does not match the LR training data with resolution $b \times a \times b$. This is the reason that the previous CNN-based SSR methods all use 2D CNNs instead of 3D CNNs.

Again, we note that current SSR methods gives the result f_1, which has improved through-plane resolution. We assume f_1 has resolution $a \times a \times c$, with $c \approx a$. Then in the second iteration, we degrade f_1 into an image with resolution $b \times a \times c$, and train a 3D network that learns the mapping from image with resolution $b \times a \times c$ to image with resolution $a \times a \times c$. The network is applied to a rotated input image g with resolution $b \times a \times a$. Although these two resolutions are not exactly the same, we believe that the trained network can tolerate this inconsistency since $c \approx a$. We iteratively perform these steps until the stop condition is met.

In this 3D iterative framework, the first iteration is SMORE using 2D networks, while the subsequent iterations use 3D networks. We designed a 3D EDSR network, with the architecture shown in Fig. 1(b). Since only the first dimension is LR, making all the convolutional kernel to be $3 \times 3 \times 3$ is a waste of parameters. We therefore only use $3 \times 3 \times 3$ kernels in the beginning and the end, while the repeated residual blocks contain $3 \times 3 \times 1$ and $3 \times 1 \times 3$ kernels. The feature number used is 256 as in 2D EDSR. Since 3D networks are more data hungry than 2D networks, we use reflection padding instead of zero padding for convolution to make good use of small training patches.

2.3   Modifications for MRI and Two-Photon Fluorescence Microscopy

The choice of 2D iSMORE or 3D iSMORE depends on the data. 3D iSMORE uses 3D CNN, which better preserves slice consistency yet is very time consuming. 2D iSMORE on the other hand, saves time and is less prone to overfitting since 2D CNNs are not as data hungry as 3D CNNs. For MRI and two-photon fluorescence microscopy, we made different modifications to iSMORE.

MRI: SMORE(3D) [10] and SMORE(2D) [11] are SSR methods designed for MRI acquired from 3D and 2D protocols. 3D MRI protocols acquire data in 3D Fourier space while 2D MRI protocols acquire data in 2D Fourier space (after slice selection). 3D MRI requires an inverse 3D Fourier transform for reconstruction while 2D MRI requires a set of inverse 2D Fourier transforms for 2D slices which are then stacked to form a 3D volume. For MRI data acquired from 3D and 2D protocols, we use corresponding SMORE as our baseline SSR method, and apply our iterative framework on SMORE, yielding iSMORE.

For further improvement, we made another modification to SMORE. The original method uses L1 loss $\sum_{\mathbf{x}} |f(\mathbf{x}) - \hat{f}(\mathbf{x})|$ to train the CNN to perform SR, with $\mathbf{x}$ being the coordinates, $\hat{f}$ being the output of the network, and f being the ground truth images. In this paper, we use a Sobel filter to compute edge maps of $\hat{f}$ and f to define a new loss function, which is previously used in Bei et al. [1]. The new loss function is $\sum_{\mathbf{x}} |f(\mathbf{x}) - \hat{f}(\mathbf{x})| + w|\text{Sobel} \circ f(\mathbf{x}) - \text{Sobel} \circ \hat{f}(\mathbf{x})|$, with weight $w = 1$. We will demonstrate its effect in Sect. 3.1.

Two-photon Fluorescence Microscopy: Two-photon fluorescence microscopy data are acquired in 2D, and then stacked into 3D volumes, which is a similar strategy at MRI acquired from 2D protocols. Thus we use SMORE(2D) as the baseline method, but we make two modifications. First, the spatial resolution (defined as the FWHM of the PSF) in the z-axis of two-photon fluorescence microscopy data is affected by the optical setting and imaging parameters. Ideally, when the laser is perfectly focused, the PSF has a closed form model, which depends on the numerical aperture (NA) of the optical system and the wavelength of the laser used [2]. However, the ideal PSF is often unable to be achieved in reality. Fortunately, we know that the orthogonal cross-section of the vessels are close to isotropic circles, and the truth isotropic HR image should have same property. Taking advantage of this fact, we can manually estimate the FWHM of PSF from those enlongated orthogonal cross-sections in the subject image by computing the fraction between the width and height of these cross-sections. We model PSF on z-axis as $Asinc(\beta z/4)^4$ [2], with β computed from the estimated FWHM.

Second, two-photon fluorescence microscopy data have a much higher noise level than MRI. An example is shown in the first column of Fig. 3. SR networks sharpen edges but also emphasize noise. To prevent further noise amplification, we add noise to the LR training data but not to the HR data, thus forcing the network to perform resolution enhancement and noise reduction at the same time. The noise we add contains both Poisson noise and speckle noise to mimic that seen in the LR subject image without noise reduction.

Finally, the two-photon fluorescence microscopy we are studying contains a large number of vessels that pass through planes and the 2D network is not able to capture enough 3D information. Therefore, we use 3D iSMORE applied to the denoised version of SMORE(2D). The 3D network uses the 3D Sobel edge loss.

3 Experiments

3.1 2D iSMORE on MRI from 3D Protocols

We compare 2D iSMORE to the original SMORE(3D) [10] using MRI down-sampled following 3D protocols. The ground truth HR images are T_2-weighted images from 14 multiple sclerosis subjects imaged on a 3T Philips Achieva scanner with acquired resolution of $1 \times 1 \times 1$ mm. The high frequency signals in z-axis are completely zeroed out to simulate 3D protocols. An additional Fermi filter is applied to simulate an anti-ringing filter. The blurred LR images have resolution $1 \times 1 \times r$ mm, where factor $r = \{2, \ldots, 6\}$. They are used as input images for methods including zero filling interpolation, SMORE(3D) [10], iSMORE with i= $\{1, \ldots, 5\}$ using SMORE (3D) as a baseline method.

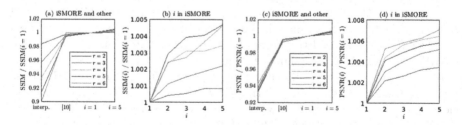

Fig. 2. SSIM and PSNR results for different anisotropic ratios r. **(a)** Ratio of the mean SSIM for zero filling interpolation, original SMORE [10], iSMORE with $i = 1$, and iSMORE with $i = 5$ with respect to iSMORE with $i = 1$. **(b)** The ratio of mean SSIM between iSMORE with $i = 1, \ldots, 5$ and $i = 1$. **(c)** Same plot as (a) for PSNR. **(d)** Same plot as (b) for PSNR

We computed Peak Signal to Noise Ratio (PSNR) and the Structural SIMilarity (SSIM) for the results of these methods using the ground truth HR images as references. The mean values are shown in Fig. 2(a) and (c). Note that the only difference between '[10]' and '$i = 1$' is that our proposed iSMORE with $i = 1$ uses the Sobel edge loss, while '[10]' does not. We see that the both the Sobel edge loss and the iterative strategy of iSMORE always improves the mean SSIM and PSNR. To show the significance of the improvement, we performed paired two-tail Wilcoxon signed-rank tests for SSIM and PSNR values between each pair of adjacent methods in Fig. 2(a) and (c), with $p = 0.005$. The significance of improvement holds everywhere except for a single case in SSIM between '[10]' and '$i = 1$' for $r = 6$.

In Fig. 2(b) and (d), we show the same ratios as in (a) and (c) but this time for the first five iterations of iSMORE. We see that greatest improvement happens between $i = 1$ and $i = 2$. If time cost is an important concern, then $i = 2$ is a good choice. Another finding is that generally the improvement from the iterative framework is larger when the LR factor r is larger. Since there is randomness including random initialization during CNN training, this finding is not strict, yet holds true in general. A third observation is that the improvement of PSNR is larger than SSIM. This might comes from the fact that the first step in computing SSIM is to apply a Gaussian filter, which degrades the details.

3.2   3D iSMORE on Two-Photon Fluorescence Microscopy

We used serial two-photon tomography (STPT) to image brain blood vessel images at cellular resolution in mice. To label blood vessel, a mouse was transcardially perfused with 0.9% saline followed by 4% paraformaldehyde and a Fluorescein isothiocyanate (FITC)-albumin conjugated gel. Detailed information about STPT imaging was described in Ragan et al. [5]. Briefly, the brain was embedded in 4% oxidized agarose and the embedded brain was placed on the motorized stage in tissuecyte 1000 (Tissuevision). The brain was imaged at 1 μm (xy-plane) resolution with 5 μm z-axis increment for 200 μm thickness.

In Fig. 3, we show the original LR image, and results of cubic b-spline interpolation (BSP), Content-AwaRE image restoration (CARE) [9] and SMORE(2D) [11] with estimated z-axis FWHM of 15 μm, the denoised version of SMORE(2D), and the proposed 3D iSMORE after the third iteration. CARE [9] is a SSR tool designed for fluorescence microscopy with a denoise option, and has publicly available code. Compared with the original LR image, BSP result has less noise and is blurry. The CARE result is sharp and relatively clean, yet many cross-sections of vessels in it are not ellipses, which implies that CARE contains sharp artifacts. The SMORE result is much sharper than BSP, but is very noisy. The denoised version of SMORE assumes Poisson noise and 30% speckle noise as described in Sect. 2.3, yielding result with much less noise, which forms our first iteration. In the second and third iterations, we train the 3D EDSR from the results of last iteration and apply it to the BSP image. The result of the proposed 3D iSMORE has vessels with more isotropic cross-sections, and contains the fewest artifacts in this comparison.

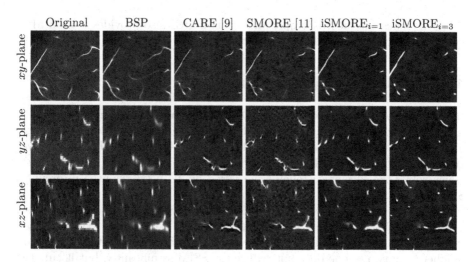

Fig. 3. Views from three orthogonal planes of the original LR image, the cubic B-spline (BSP) interpolated image, result of CARE [9], SMORE(2D) [11], our denoised version of SMORE(2D) which is also the first iteration of iSMORE, and our proposed 3D iSMORE with $i = 3$

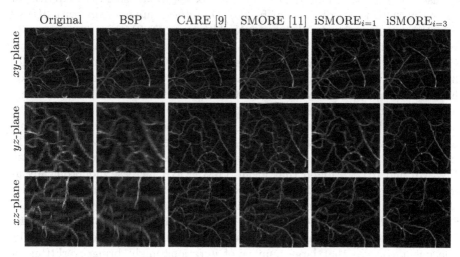

Fig. 4. Maximum intensity projection (MIP) on three orthogonal planes of the original LR image, the cubic B-spline (BSP) interpolated image, result of CARE [9], SMORE(2D) [11], our denoise version of SMORE(2D) which is also the first iteration of iSMORE, and our proposed 3D iSMORE with $i = 3$

It is very difficult to obtain isotropic HR ground truth for STPT data since owning laser device with isotropic PSF is not common. Thus metrics like SSIM and PSNR are not available. In order to show its overall performance in the 3D volume, we perform maximum intensity projection (MIP) on three planes, and show the MIP results in Fig. 4. Visually, the MIP of the proposed method iSMORE looks the most isotropic and clear. CARE also provides a good MIP, yet the artifacts shown in Fig. 3 cannot be ignored.

4   Conclusion and Discussion

In this paper, we described 2D and 3D iSMORE, an iterative framework built upon the SMORE method. The idea behind iSMORE is that thick in-plane slices are not as good training data as thin slices. Using this idea, iSMORE improves the performance of SMORE. And more importantly, it enables a 3D network, which solves the slice consistency issue raised by 2D networks used in previous SSR methods.

There are some details of iSMORE that we would like to discuss. First, we used SMORE with only one orientation, while the original SMORE used two orientations [10,11]. In practice, we found that reducing the orientation number from two to one does not reduce the SSIM significantly, but it cuts the computation time in half. This strategy is also adopted by another paper from the author of SMORE [12]. Future work will include a more detailed exploration on the choice of number of orientations. Second, it might be confusing that we use 2D iSMORE for images with 3D protocols, while using 3D iSMORE for images with 2D protocols. To clarify, 2D/3D protocols are not same with 2D/3D iSMORE, which refers to 2D/3D CNN. Although 3D iSMORE preserves slice consistency, 2D iSMORE uses a 2D CNN, is easier to train, and saves time. One more iteration takes about 20 mins for 2D iSMORE, and more than 1 h for 3D iSMORE on microscopy data. Images acquired with 3D protocols already have good slice consistency, so 2D iSMORE is able to handle them. For images acquired with 2D protocols, slice consistency is more of a concern. Thus, 3D iSMORE is a better choice in this case, with the penalty of larger compute time. Third, the number of iterations of iSMORE in this paper is manually set. To clarify, due to time cost, we do not recommend a large number of iterations. From Fig. 2(b) and (d), we found that mean SSIM/PSNR increase monotonically as iteration i increases from 1 to 5. However, we only recommend use of $i = 2$ for this dataset since time increases linearly with i. For microscopy data, we use $i = 3$ since the improvement between the 2nd and 3rd iteration is still large. Future work will include a more detailed discussion on the choice of i. Finally, one might concern that large number of iterations might bring overfitting or artifacts. However from our experiment, in Fig. 2, both SSIM/PSNR increase with iteration count; while in Fig. 3, iSMORE with $i = 3$ has better cross-sectional shapes and fewer artifacts than iSMORE with $i = 1$ and CARE which also uses only one iteration.

In summary, we describe a new algorithm iSMORE in this paper, we evaluated it both quantitatively and qualitatively, and experimented with it on both downsampled and real acquired low resolution medical images with two very different modalities. We applied iSMORE to downsampled MR images with ground truth HR images to evaluate its accuracy with SSIM and PSNR. The results show that both Sobel edge loss and the iterative framework can significantly improve the accuracy. Furthermore, we adjusted iSMORE for real-world acquired two-photon fluorescence microscopy data which have a higher noise level and more 3D information than MRI. The result and its maximum intensity projection on three orthogonal planes are visually more isotropic, the vessels are visually clearer and easier to track than the original SMORE. Future work will include a deeper exploration on the parameters used in this algorithm as well as a comparison on different network architectures.

Acknowledgments. This work was supported by the NIH under grant R01-NS108407, R01-NS105503, and the National Multiple Sclerosis Society grant RG-1507-05243. Thanks to Aaron Carass for valuable discussion.

References

1. Bei, Y., Damian, A., Hu, S., Menon, S., Ravi, N., Rudin, C.: New techniques for preserving global structure and denoising with low information loss in single-image super-resolution. In: Proceedings of the IEEE Conference on Computer Vision and Pattern Recognition Workshops, pp. 874–881 (2018)
2. Helmchen, F., Denk, W.: Deep tissue two-photon microscopy. Nat. Methods 2(12), 932 (2005)
3. Jog, A., Carass, A., Prince, J.L.: Self super-resolution for magnetic resonance images. In: Ourselin, S., Joskowicz, L., Sabuncu, M.R., Unal, G., Wells, W. (eds.) MICCAI 2016. LNCS, vol. 9902, pp. 553–560. Springer, Cham (2016). https://doi.org/10.1007/978-3-319-46726-9_64
4. Lim, B., Son, S., Kim, H., Nah, S., Mu Lee, K.: Enhanced deep residual networks for single image super-resolution. In: Proceedings of the IEEE Conference on Computer Vision and Pattern Recognition Workshops, pp. 136–144 (2017)
5. Ragan, T., et al.: Serial two-photon tomography for automated ex vivo mouse brain imaging. Nat. Methods 9(3), 255 (2012)
6. Ronneberger, O., Fischer, P., Brox, T.: U-Net: convolutional networks for biomedical image segmentation. In: Navab, N., Hornegger, J., Wells, W.M., Frangi, A.F. (eds.) MICCAI 2015. LNCS, vol. 9351, pp. 234–241. Springer, Cham (2015). https://doi.org/10.1007/978-3-319-24574-4_28
7. Timofte, R., De Smet, V., Van Gool, L.: Anchored neighborhood regression for fast example-based super-resolution. In: Proceedings of the IEEE International Conference on Computer Vision, pp. 1920–1927 (2013)
8. Timofte, R., Gu, S., Wu, J., Van Gool, L.: Ntire 2018 challenge on single image super-resolution: methods and results. In: Proceedings of the IEEE Conference on Computer Vision and Pattern Recognition Workshops, pp. 852–863 (2018)
9. Weigert, M., et al.: Content-aware image restoration: pushing the limits of fluorescence microscopy. Nat. Methods 15(12), 1090 (2018)
10. Zhao, C., Carass, A., Dewey, B.E., Prince, J.L.: Self super-resolution for magnetic resonance images using deep networks. In: IEEE International Symposium on Biomedical Imaging (ISBI) (2018)
11. Zhao, C., et al.: A deep learning based anti-aliasing self super-resolution algorithm for MRI. In: Frangi, A.F., Schnabel, J.A., Davatzikos, C., Alberola-López, C., Fichtinger, G. (eds.) MICCAI 2018. LNCS, vol. 11070, pp. 100–108. Springer, Cham (2018). https://doi.org/10.1007/978-3-030-00928-1_12
12. Zhao, C., et al.: Applications of a deep learning method for anti-aliasing and super-resolution in MRI. Magnetic Resonance Imaging (2019)

An Optical Model of Whole Blood for Detecting Platelets in Lens-Free Images

Benjamin D. Haeffele[1]($\boxtimes$) , Christian Pick[1], Ziduo Lin[2], Evelien Mathieu[1], Stuart C. Ray[1] , and René Vidal[1]

[1] Johns Hopkins University, Baltimore, MD, USA
bhaeffele@jhu.edu
[2] Imec, Leuven, Belgium

Abstract. In this paper we consider the task of detecting platelets in images of diluted whole blood taken with a lens-free microscope. Despite having several advantages over traditional microscopes, lens-free imaging systems have the significant challenge that the resolution of the system is typically limited by the pixel dimensions of the image sensor. As a result of this limited resolution, detecting platelets is very difficult to do even by manual inspection of the images due to the fact that platelets occupy just a few pixels of the reconstructed image. To address this challenge, we develop an optical model of diluted whole blood to generate physically realistic simulated holograms which we then use to train a convolutional neural network (CNN) for platelet detection. We validate our approach by collecting both lens-free and fluorescent microscopy images of the same field of view of diluted whole blood samples with fluorescently labeled platelets.

Keywords: Lens-free imaging · Holography · Object detection

1 Introduction

Lens-free imaging (LFI) is a form of digital microscopic holography which records the diffraction patterns (also referred to as holograms) of a specimen illuminated with coherent light (e.g., from a laser) and then reconstructs an image of the specimen by inverting a mathematical model of the light diffraction process. LFI has multiple advantages over conventional microscopy. First, as the name implies, the system does not require lenses which significantly reduces the overall system cost, complexity, and size. Second, LFI systems have larger fields of view than traditional microscopes with equivalent magnification. Third, the system does not require any manual focusing as the focal depth can be adjusted via software, which additionally eliminates the strict mechanical stability requirements of lens-based systems (where the lens must be held at a precise focal distance from the image sensor) [4].

Here, we are interested in exploiting these advantages of LFI systems to develop a compact and low-cost system that is capable of measuring the concentration of platelets in human blood. Platelet counts are an indispensable tool in

© Springer Nature Switzerland AG 2019
N. Burgos et al. (Eds.): SASHIMI 2019, LNCS 11827, pp. 140–150, 2019.
https://doi.org/10.1007/978-3-030-32778-1_15

modern medicine and make up one of the standard analytes of a complete blood count (CBC), one of the most widely ordered blood tests worldwide. Additionally, abnormal platelet counts can indicate a wide variety of pathologies, and many clinical situations require routine monitoring of platelet counts. However, despite the previously mentioned advantages of LFI systems and the significant clinical need for monitoring platelet counts, a significant challenge in LFI applications is that the resolution of LFI systems is often limited by the pixel size of the image sensor (typically around 1 micron square for common commercial grade sensors). A platelet typically has a diameter of only 2–3 microns and a volume of only 9–12 femtoliters, making identification of platelets in reconstructed LFI images very challenging even with close manual inspection of the image. As an example, Fig. 1 (Middle) shows a small crop from a reconstructed image of diluted whole blood. Note that while some platelets are visible (a few are denoted with red arrows), they are hard to identify manually and can be easily confused with artifacts in the reconstructed image (the full, uncropped image can be found in the supplement).

Current state-of-the-art systems for object detection in images are all largely based on deep neural networks (see [3,7,8] for a few well-known examples). However, training large network models requires access to significant volumes of training images along with corresponding ground-truth regarding the location of the various objects of interest. As described above, it is often very challenging to accurately locate and identify platelets in reconstructed lens-free images due to their small size relative to the resolution of the image and the relatively small signal that they generate relative to the other cells in the image (predominately red blood cells), which limits the potential of constructing large training sets.

In this work, we address these challenges by developing an optical model which allows us to simulate synthetic holograms of diluted whole blood with sufficient realism to train a convolutional neural network (CNN) capable of detecting platelets in real LFI images. In addition, to validate our approach we also constructed a tandem microscopy imaging setup which allows us to record an LFI hologram and a fluorescent image of an overlapping field-of-view within a few seconds of each other. By fluorescently labeling platelets we then compare the platelet detections from our trained neural network operating on LFI images with detections from the corresponding fluorescent image (which is much easier due to the fluorescent labeling).

2 Optical Model

To develop our optical model of diluted whole blood, we need a means to optically model the various cell types present in human blood: red blood cells (RBCs), platelets (PLTs), and white blood cells (WBCs). WBCs are relatively uncommon (roughly 3 orders of magnitude lower concentrations than RBCs), so their presence or absence in an image has little impact on detecting PLTs. As a result, we will largely focus on modeling RBCs and PLTs.

Red Blood Cell Model. To model the optical properties of an RBC, we use a phase-plate model which describes the modulation of the incident light wave that is created by the RBC as a phase shift proportional to the integration of the RBC shape along the optical axis (by common convention we'll use the z axis as the direction of light propagation). This model is consistent with scattering measurements taken of RBCs which have also noted that at the wavelength of light used by our LFI system (637 nm) RBCs do not absorb light [2]. With this model, the optical modulation of the incident wavefront is entirely determined by the RBC shape and orientation (and more specifically the integral of the shape along the optical axis), so to model the RBC shape, we use the parametric model for RBC shape given in [5], which takes the general form:

$$(x^2 + y^2 + z^2)^2 + P(x^2 + y^2) + Qz^2 + R \leq 0, \tag{1}$$

where (P, Q, R) are coefficients determined by the minimum thickness of the RBC, h_{min}, the maximal thickness of the RBC, h_{max}, and the diameter of the RBC, d, given as:

$$P = \tfrac{1}{2}\left[-d^2 + h_{max}^2\left((\tfrac{d}{h_{min}})^2 - 1\right)\left(1 - \sqrt{1 - (\tfrac{h_{min}}{h_{max}})^2}\right)\right]$$
$$R = -(\tfrac{d}{2})^2 P - (\tfrac{d}{2})^4 \qquad Q = (\tfrac{d}{h_{min}})^2 P + (\tfrac{h_{min}}{2})^2((\tfrac{d}{h_{min}})^4 - 1). \tag{2}$$

Given the general shape of an RBC (see Fig. 1 (Left) for an illustration of the relevant dimensions), we then generate RBCs at arbitrary orientations and locations in the image by rotating and translating the coordinate system in (1) for each RBC and then integrate along the optical axis to produce the total path length image (path length is proportional to phase shift) induced by the kth RBC as:

$$\bar{\theta}_k^{RBC}(x, y) = \int \mathbb{I}[(\bar{x}_k^2 + \bar{y}_k^2 + \bar{z}_k^2)^2 + P_k(\bar{x}_k^2 + \bar{y}_k^2) + Q_k\bar{z}_k^2 + R_k \leq 0]dz, \tag{3}$$

where $\mathbb{I}[c]$ is an indicator function which takes value 1 if condition c is true and 0 otherwise, $(\bar{x}_k, \bar{y}_k, \bar{z}_k)$ are the rotated and translated coordinates for the kth RBC, and (P_k, Q_k, R_k) are the coefficients for RBC k with a prescribed set of shape dimensions $(d_k, h_{max,k}, h_{min,k})$, each independently sampled for each cell uniformly over the ranges $([7, 8.5], [2, 2.5], [0.8, 1.4])\mu$m, respectively.

Platelet Model. Since platelets are very small for the resolution of images we are simulating, we use a very simple model for them in our simulations as additional details will be largely irrelevant after image discretization. Namely, we again assume that platelets modulate the light wavefront largely by simply shifting the phase of the wavefront (i.e., they do not significantly absorb light). As a result, we model platelets as being a simple disk of shifted phase

$$\theta_j^{PLT}(x, y) = \psi_j \mathbb{I}[\bar{x}_j^2 + \bar{y}_j^2 \leq r_j^2], \tag{4}$$

where ψ_j denotes a constant phase shift (which we uniformly sample from $[0.25, 0.75]/(2\pi)$ radians based on typical measurements of platelets in our reconstructed images) applied to all pixels within platelet j, where $(\bar{x}_j, \bar{y}_j)$ are the

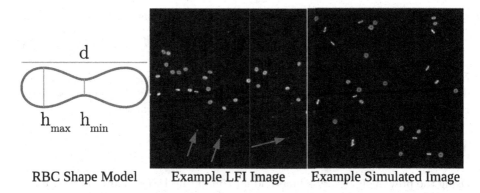

RBC Shape Model Example LFI Image Example Simulated Image

Fig. 1. (Left) Parameters of the RBC shape model. (Middle) Small crop of an example reconstructed LFI image. Red arrows denote example platelets. (Right) Small crop from an example reconstructed image from our simulator. (Color figure online)

translated coordinates for the jth platelet, and r_j is the radius of the jth platelet, sampled uniformly over the range $[0.8, 1.5]\,\mu m$.

Full Model. Given these individual models for both PLTs and RBCs, we then simulate the (complex valued) optical wavefront at the image plane by combining the various phase shifts induced by all the simulated cells of various sizes, locations, and orientations:

$$I(x,y) = \exp\left\{2\pi i\left[\frac{\nu_{RBC} - \nu_{media}}{\lambda}\sum_k \bar{\theta}_k^{RBC}(x,y) + \sum_j \theta_j^{PLT}(x,y)\right]\right\}, \quad (5)$$

where $\nu_{RBC} = 1.4$ is the refractive index of an RBC at our illumination wavelength, $\lambda = 637\,nm$, as measured in [2], and $\nu_{media} = 1.33$ is the refractive index of the fluid media suspending the blood cells.

Given the simulated wavefront at the image plane, $I(x,y)$, we then simulate the hologram by projecting the wavefront at the specimen plane to the image sensor plane a distance z_0 away (we sample uniformly over $[400, 1200]\,\mu m$ in our simulations) using the wide-angular spectrum (WAS) model for light propagation [4] which projects the wavefront via a convolution with a transfer function $I_{z_0}(x,y) = t_{z_0}(x,y) * I(x,y)$, with the transfer function, $t_{z_0}(x,y)$, defined in Fourier space as,

$$\mathcal{F}\left\{t_{z_0}(x,y)\right\}[k_x, k_y] = \exp\left(iz_0\sqrt{(\tfrac{2\pi}{\lambda})^2 - k_x^2 - k_y^2}\right). \quad (6)$$

Once the simulated wavefront is projected to the image sensor plane, we then produce a final simulated hologram by taking the absolute value of the wavefront due to the physics of the image sensor only being able to record the magnitude of the optical wavefront but not the phase. Finally, we add a small amount of sampling noise, to produce the final simulated hologram as follows,

$$H(x,y) = |I_{z_0}(x,y)| + \epsilon(x,y) \quad \text{where} \quad \epsilon(x,y) \overset{i.i.d.}{\sim} \mathcal{N}(0,\sigma) \ \forall(x,y). \quad (7)$$

Here we have used a Gaussian noise model for the image sensor, with standard deviations uniform over the range $[0.0125, 0.03125]$, but other noise models (e.g., Poisson) could also be employed depending on the application.

3   Platelet Detection

Using the previously described method for simulating LFI holograms, we trained a convolutional neural network (CNN) to detect platelet locations from the recorded hologram. The first step in this process is to reconstruct an image of the specimen from the simulated hologram, for which we employ the sparse phase recovery reconstruction method developed in [1]. Figure 1 shows example reconstructions from both a real hologram and a simulated hologram, which have strong qualitative similarities. In addition to sensor noise added to the simulated hologram, we also add an offset (uniformly sampled over $\pm 3\,\mu\text{m}$) to the reconstruction focal depth versus the true focal depth used to generate the simulated hologram to account for potential errors in auto-focusing that can occur when reconstructing real images. After reconstruction, the image is complex valued, representing an estimate of the image wavefront at the specimen plane (all images of reconstructions show the absolute value of the wavefront), so to train a CNN to detect platelets, we split the real and imaginary components of the reconstruction into two input channels to the network. The rest of the network is then a fully convolutional network, consisting of a sequence of six convolutional layers with kernels of spatial dimension 3×3 and the number of output channels reducing by a factor of 2 each layer ($[32, 16, 8, 4, 2, 1]$, respectively). Rectified Linear Unit (ReLU) non-linearities are applied entry-wise after each convolution, with the exception of the final layer which applies a sigmoid non-linearity (a diagram of the network architecture can be found in the supplement). The use of a fully convolutional network was done for two reasons. First, it allows the network to be applied to an input image of arbitrary size, and second, due to the small size of the platelets in these images we did not want to lose any spatial information regarding their location through any operation that reduces the image dimension (such as max-pooling).

Note that the output of the network is an image with the same spatial dimension as the input, where the magnitude of each pixel is the probability that the pixel contains a platelet. As a result, we train the network as a pixel-wise classification problem using the cross-entropy loss applied pixel-wise comparing to whether a given pixel contains a platelet in the simulated image. The network weights are optimized using standard stochastic gradient descent with Nesterov acceleration. Mini-batches of 10 simulated images with dimension 1024×1024 are generated, and for each mini-batch 50 gradient descent steps are taken before a new mini-batch is generated. To perform inference on unseen real images, we simply threshold the output image at a value of 0.5 (recall the sigmoid non-linearity outputs a value in the range $[0, 1]$) and treat each connected component in the thresholded image as a platelet detection with no morphological filtering.

4   Testing and Validation

The fact that PLTs are very hard to detect even manually in LFI images presents significant challenges not only to the training of PLT detection methods (as discussed above) but also to the testing and validation of such methods as one often does not have access to high quality ground truth information. To address this issue, we developed a tandem microscopy setup which allows for both fluorescent and LFI images with a partially overlapping field of view (FOV) to be recorded within a few seconds of each other. By fluorescently labeling the PLTs (we use a CD41/CD61-FITC human antibody label from Miltenyi Biotec) we can then detect PLTs in the fluorescent images with fairly high confidence (as they are the only fluorescent objects in the image), and we then compare the set of detections in the fluorescent images with those in the LFI images.

PLT Detection in Fluorescent Images. To detect the fluorescently labeled PLTs in the fluorescent images we perform a standard image denoising procedure based on sparse dictionary learning [6], where we first extract all 10×10 pixel patches from the image using a sliding window, normalize the patches to have zero mean and unit Euclidean norm, train a sparse dictionary from the patches, reconstruct the patches using a sparse encoding approximation with the learned dictionary, and finally regenerate the denoised image by returning the patches to the appropriate locations and averaging over the overlapping patches. Once the fluorescent images have been denoised via dictionary learning, the platelets are easily detected via a simple thresholding. The middle column of Fig. 2 shows an example image of the denoised fluorescent image and corresponding detections (the dots indicate a detection in the fluorescent image, and the color of the dot indicates whether the corresponding PLT was detected in the LFI image). The original fluorescent image is given in Fig. 5.

Aligning Fluorescent and LFI Images. Once PLT detection has been performed on both an LFI image and a corresponding fluorescent image, we then align the coordinate systems between the two image modalities. Although the two image modalities have a partially overlapping FOV, the two images are taken at different magnifications and spatial offsets relative to each other, so to register the two sets of image coordinates we fit an affine transformation using an alternating minimization approach where we begin with a rough estimate of the alignment transformation between the images. Then, given the assumed alignment, we project one set of PLT detections into the coordinates of the other set and match the two sets of detections using a linear assignment with an Euclidean distance cost to produce correspondences. Using the new proposed assignments we then update the parameters of the affine transformation between the coordinate systems to minimize the Euclidean error between the proposed correspondences between the two sets of detections.

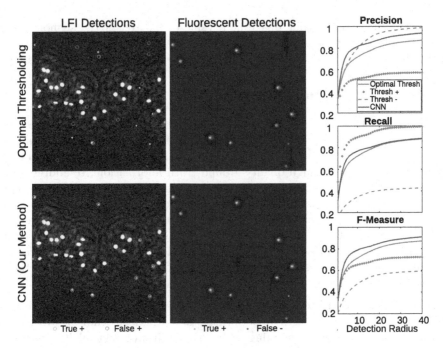

Fig. 2. (Left) Example detections from our method (bottom row) and an optimal thresholding baseline (top row). The left column shows the LFI image from the previous figure (with a saturated gray-scale to better visualize PLTs). The right column shows the corresponding denoised fluorescent image after alignment to the LFI coordinate system. Green circles (LFI Image) and dots (fluorescent image) denote true detections where the LFI detection matched a fluorescent detection (using a detection radius of 10 pixels). Red circles (LFI Image) denote false positive detections in the LFI image, and Red dots (fluorescent image) denote false negatives (a detection in the fluorescent image that was not detected in the LFI image). (Right) Precision, Recall, and F-Measure values as a function of detection radius. (Color figure online)

Performance Metrics and Baselines. To evaluate the performance of our combined model (a PLT detection CNN trained using images from our simulator) we collected a dataset of 39 paired images consisting of both LFI and fluorescent images. We then treat the PLT detections in the fluorescent image as a ground truth and compute precision and recall scores along with the F-measure (the F-measure is defined as $2(precision * recall)/(precision + recall)$). Due to the fact that the LFI and fluorescent images are not collected at exactly the same time, the cells (which are suspended in a microfluidic flow-cell channel) can move slightly between image acquisitions, so even after the coordinate set alignment described above there is still some offset between detections in the two image modalities. As a result, we compute the precision, recall, and F-measure statistics as a function of an allowed detection radius, where we label a detection in the LFI image as being correct if it is within the detection radius of a detection in the fluorescent image. Specifically, we solve a linear assignment problem between the two sets of detections (LFI and fluorescent), with zero cost in matching two detections if they lie within the detection radius of each other and a cost of one if they lie outside of that radius. Any detections lying outside the overlapping FOV between the two images (after coordinate alignment) were discarded.

To compare our method against a baseline, the fact that in our original problem we do not have knowledge of ground truth locations again presents difficulty as we cannot compare against any supervised approaches for object detection. As a result, we use an "optimal" thresholding baseline, where we study the best performance that can be achieved via simple thresholding. Specifically, we threshold the LFI image and then label a connected component in the thresholded image a PLT if its area is within lower and upper bound limits. We then maximize the F-measure at a detection radius of 25 pixels by performing an exhaustive grid search over the choice of the image intensity threshold and lower/upper bounds on the connected component area. Note that this uses full knowledge of the ground-truth to tune the thresholding hyperparameters and as a result is an over-estimate of the performance of thresholding. Figure 2 (right column) shows that even though the optimal thresholding method makes full use of the ground-truth in selecting hyperparameters our method still achieves a higher F-measure across all choices of allowed detection radii. Additionally, the optimal thresholding method is very unstable to choice of hyperparameters, and simply increasing (Thresh +) or decreasing (Thresh −) the upper and lower limits of the connected component area by the minimum increment in the grid search (3 pixels) significantly degrades performance. Further, manual examination of the detection locations in the top left of Fig. 2 shows that thresholding (even with optimal choice of thresholding hyperparameters) produces poor detections that qualitatively do not correspond to the true platelet locations. In contrast our CNN, trained using our developed optical simulator, achieves very good qualitative performance for the platelets that can be observed by eye and over 80% F-Measure score once the detection radius is above approximately 10 pixels, roughly on the order of the alignment error between the LFI and fluorescent coordinates due to cells drifting between the two image acquisitions.

5   Conclusions

We have presented an optical model of diluted whole blood that is sufficiently realistic to be successful in training a CNN based object detection network. Our approach achieves good performance on the very difficult task of detecting platelets in reconstructed LFI images, which can be challenging even by manual inspection due to the limited resolution of LFI systems and additionally presents significant challenges in even validating a given method. As a result, to validate our approach we developed and constructed a tandem microscopy setup which allows for close to simultaneous imaging of a fluorescent image (with fluorescently labeled platelets) and a LFI image of an overlapping field of view.

Acknowledgments. This work was funded by miDiagnostics.

Supplemental Figures

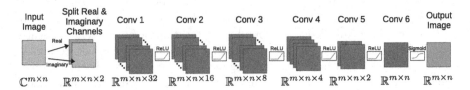

Fig. 3. Network architecture used for platelet detection. The first step is to convert the complex-valued input image into a real-valued tensor by splitting the real and imaginary values at each pixel into two separate channels. The remaining network is then fully convolutional with bias terms with ReLU non-linearities following each convolution with the exception of the final convolution which uses a sigmoid non-linearity. Every convolutional kernel used a spatial dimension of 3×3 with a stride of 1. The indicated dimensions correspond to the output dimension of the representation following the convolution of that layer (e.g., the output of the Conv 1 layer is $m \times n \times 32$). Layers in blue contain trainable parameters. (Color figure online)

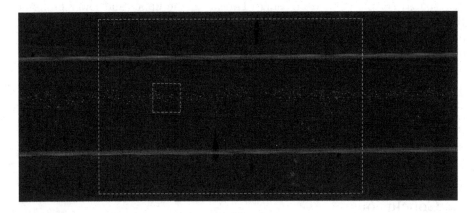

Fig. 4. The full reconstructed LFI image used to generate the example crops in the main paper. (Red dashed square) Region shown in the main paper. (Yellow dashed rectangle) Field of view that is overlapping with the fluorescent image (see Fig. 5). The horizontal lines in the image that run the full width the image are the walls of the microfluidic channel. (Color figure online)

Fig. 5. (Top) The raw fluorescent image used to generate the fluorescent images in the main paper. (Bottom) The fluorescent image following the sparse dictionary learning denoising (all fluorescent images shown in the main paper are following denoising). For both images, the dashed red square indicates the region used to show the example crops in the main paper. The horizontal lines in the image that run the full width the image are the walls of the microfluidic channel. (Color figure online)

References

1. Haeffele, B.D., Stahl, R., Vanmeerbeeck, G., Vidal, R.: Efficient reconstruction of holographic lens-free images by sparse phase recovery. In: Descoteaux, M., Maier-Hein, L., Franz, A., Jannin, P., Collins, D.L., Duchesne, S. (eds.) MICCAI 2017. LNCS, vol. 10434, pp. 109–117. Springer, Cham (2017). https://doi.org/10.1007/978-3-319-66185-8_13
2. Hammer, M., Schweitzer, D., Michel, B., Thamm, E., Kolb, A.: Single scattering by red blood cells. Appl. Opt. **37**(31), 7410–7418 (1998)
3. He, K., Gkioxari, G., Dollár, P., Girshick, R.: Mask R-CNN. In: IEEE International Conference on Computer Vision, pp. 2961–2969 (2017)
4. Kim, M.K.: Digital Holographic Microscopy. Springer, New York (2011). https://doi.org/10.1007/978-1-4419-7793-9
5. Kuchel, P.W., Fackerell, E.D.: Parametric-equation representation of biconcave erythrocytes. Bull. Math. Biol. **61**(2), 209–220 (1999)
6. Mairal, J., Bach, F., Ponce, J., Sapiro, G.: Online learning for matrix factorization and sparse coding. J. Mach. Learn. Res. **11**, 19–60 (2010)
7. Redmon, J., Divvala, S., Girshick, R., Farhadi, A.: You only look once: unified, real-time object detection. In: IEEE Conference on Computer Vision and Pattern Recognition, pp. 779–788 (2016)
8. Ren, S., He, K., Girshick, R., Sun, J.: Faster R-CNN: towards real-time object detection with region proposal networks. In: Neural Information Processing Systems, pp. 91–99 (2015)

Evaluation of the Realism of an MRI Simulator for Stroke Lesion Prediction Using Convolutional Neural Network

Noëlie Debs[1], Méghane Decroocq[1], Tae-Hee Cho[1], David Rousseau[2], and Carole Frindel[1](✉)

[1] CREATIS, CNRS UMR-5220, INSERM U1206, Université Lyon 1, INSA Lyon, 7 avenue Jean Capelle, 69621 Villeurbanne, France
`carole.frindel@creatis.insa-lyon.fr`
[2] LARIS, UMR IRHS INRA, Université d'Angers, 62 avenue Notre Dame du Lac, 49000 Angers, France

Abstract. We are focusing on the difficult task of predicting final lesion in stroke, a complex disease that leads to divergent imaging patterns related to the occluded artery level and the geometry of the patient's vascular tree. We propose a framework in which convolutional neural networks are trained only from synthetic perfusion MRI - obtained from an existing physical simulator - and tested on real patients. We incorporate new levels of realism into this simulator, allowing to simulate the vascular tree of a given patient. We demonstrate that our approach is able to predict the final infarct of the tested patients only from simulated data. Among the various simulated databases generated, we show that simulations taking into account the vascular tree information give the best classification performances on the tested patients.

Keywords: Perfusion MRI · Lesion prediction · Simulation · Arterial input function · Time of transport · Convolutional neural network

1 Introduction

Stroke is the leading cause of long-term disability and mortality worldwide. Ischemic stroke (85% of all stroke cases) results from an acute occlusion of a cerebral artery. Acute neuroimaging is crucial to choose the best therapeutic option [4] and in particular to understand the lesion evolution. One commonly used imaging modality for acute stroke patient management is perfusion MRI, obtained by the acquisition of a dynamic MRI sequence synchronized with the intravenous injection of a contrast-agent. Perfusion MRI produces a temporal concentration signal recorded in each voxel of a volume of interest. After deconvolution, these signals are post-processed to obtain hemodynamic biomarkers which are used for interpretation. Lesion prediction is then addressed by thresholding these biomarkers based on kinetic models. However, the dispersion of the

© Springer Nature Switzerland AG 2019
N. Burgos et al. (Eds.): SASHIMI 2019, LNCS 11827, pp. 151–160, 2019.
https://doi.org/10.1007/978-3-030-32778-1_16

contrast agent may reflect, in addition to tissue perfusion, macrovascular properties. To overcome this problem, several deconvolution techniques have been proposed in the last decades [1,5,17]. In this context, simulation plays an important role to validate deconvolution methods by generating synthetic and annotated ground truth images and associated simulated acquired images [7,12]. Such validation is required to understand the characteristics of deconvolution methods and to evaluate their performance and limitations.

More recently, deep learning models have been successfully proposed as a way to predict lesion without deconvolution [18]. In this context, the amount of training data is critical for making supervised machine learning models accurate, especially when using algorithms which require a large number of parameters to be discriminating. A way to get around this problem is to generate more data to increase variability in the learning dataset and thus improve regularization and reduce overfitting. While simple transformations applied to existing datasets (e.g. translation, rotation) often produce highly correlated images, image synthesis from statistical or physical models appears to better supplement the training dataset, although it is more complex to achieve [15,20]. In this framework, we propose to increase the effectiveness of the simulated produced by an existing physical simulator [7] for training segmentation algorithms. This simulator, which is currently the only one that consider the spatial context of brain tissues and lesions, seemed therefore appropriate to test a new source of spatial variability related to stroke: the vascular tree. Anatomical studies have described typical configurations of the Circle of Willis (CW) [10]. In view of this large number of variations, it appears that the existence of an effective arterial CW could not always be assumed. According to [16], incompleteness of the CW or poor collateral circulation was significantly related to the embolism risk.

In this work, we propose to improve the realism of the perfusion MRI simulator proposed by [7]. This new version enables a patient-specific simulation of vascular tree anatomy. Our simulation framework consists of medical image-driven modeling of patient vascular tree through arterial flow and contrast agent time of transport modeling. A total of 8 patient-specific models were considered, with varying levels of occlusion in the brain and varying morphologies of vascular tree. The realism improvement was evaluated by training a convolutional neural network on the generated synthetic data and testing the resulting model on real data. The results were assessed using the Dice and Hausdorff metrics.

2   Methods

2.1   Clinical MRI

Clinical data are from the European I-Know multicenter database [9]. On admission, all patients underwent diffusion-weighted imaging (DWI), fluid-attenuated inversion-recovery (FLAIR), T2-weighted gradient echo, time-of-flight MR angiography, and perfusion-weighted imaging (DSC-PWI). A follow-up FLAIR-MRI was performed at 1-month after admission time. Perfusion MRI were registered, for each slice, using the first time point as reference for all the other time points, with a maximum mutual information approach. Final lesion was segmented for each patient on the 1-month follow-up FLAIR-MRI by 3 experts. FLAIR-MRI volumes were first coregistered to DSC-PWI volumes computed by avering the temporal signal before contrast-agent arrival. The transformation matrix obtained was then used to register the final ischemic lesion mask. All registrations were performed using Elastix.

We selected 8 patients from the 110 available in the I-Know cohort. They were representative of the different levels of occlusion in the middle cerebral artery (2 in M1 segment, 3 in M2 segment, 2 in M3 segment and 1 unknown) and of the different CW geometries with different number of communicating arteries (3 with 3 communications, 2 with 2 communications, 2 with 1 communication and 1 with no communication). Also they came from 2 distinct medical centers.

2.2 Description of the Perfusion MRI Simulator

We briefly recall the principle of the simulator developed by [7]. Their approach consist in generating contrast-agent concentration images by convolution between an arterial input function (AIF) and a simulated impulse response. Several input parameters are adjustable such as realistic brain and lesion shapes with distinct classes of tissues (infarcted, healthy gray matter, healthy white matter), the associated statistical distribution of hemodynamic parameters, and AIF parameters. In the simulator, AIF is modeled as a gamma function that can be expressed using the simplified formulation proposed by [14]:

$$\Gamma(t) = \begin{cases} 0, & \text{if } t \le d \\ y_{max} \cdot (\frac{t-d}{t_{max}})^\alpha \cdot \exp\left(\alpha(1 - \frac{t-d}{t_{max}})\right), & \text{if } t \ge d \end{cases}, \quad (1)$$

where y_{max} and t_{max} respectively correspond to the magnitude and position of the maximum of the AIF, d is the arrival time of the contrast agent and α corresponds to the shape parameter of the gamma function.

By default in the simulator, AIF is represented by a single global gamma function described in the literature [11] by the following parameters: $y_{max} = 0.61$, $t_{max} = 4.5$, $d = 3$, $\alpha = 3$. The simulator allows to modify these parameters to simulate patients with other specific macrovascular properties. To simulate a specific patient, it is necessary to estimate its own AIF by positioning a ROI near a major contralateral artery and then averaging the extracted signals to produce a single global AIF.

To improve the physiological realism of this simulator, we propose to model the patient-specific vascular tree anatomy. This modeling step includes arterial flow and contrast agent time of transport variations and is graphically summarized in Fig. 1.

2.3 Integration of the Arterial Flow Variability

The assumption of a global and unique AIF has recently been questioned [13] since an important AIF variability can be observed when extracting concentration signals from a major contralateral artery in the perfusion image of a specific

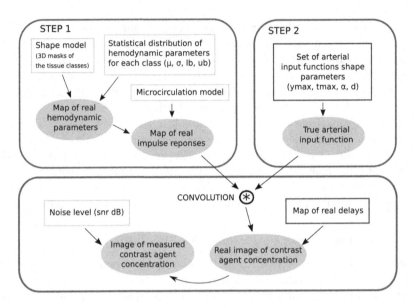

Fig. 1. Pipeline of the new version of the perfusion MRI simulator. The newly introduced sources of variability are displayed in dark blue. (Color figure online)

patient (see Fig. 2). These variations may be caused by imaging artifacts (such as partial volume effect, low temporal resolution) [6] or even the presence of stenosis causing a lower peak and wider bolus shape in the supply territory of the stenotic artery [2]. This intra-patient AIF variability has been incorporated into the new version of the proposed simulator by the integration of a set of multiple specific AIF shapes.

To this end, we first used patient data to characterize its AIF range and associated parameters. These are then given as input to the simulator which represents the 4 AIF parameters in a 4D space (each axis representing a parameter of Eq. 1) and computes a Delaunay triangulation. Finally, the set of multiple specific AIF shapes was produced by a random selection in the associated 4D Delaunay polygon.

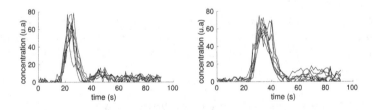

Fig. 2. Set of manually extracted AIFs (black) and its associated median signal (red) for 2 patients of our study. For illustration, intra-patient AIF variability is greater on the right than on the left. (Color figure online)

2.4   Integration of the Contrast Agent Time of Transport

The transport of contrast agent along the vascular tree results in an increasing delay (i.e temporal shift) of the AIF in the periphery of the brain [3]. Taking into account this phenomena in the simulation would enable to reach a new degree of spatial realism and might provide important information about the vascular supply of the lesion, and eventual collateral flow (alternate circulation around a blocked artery). This could have consequences on the geometry of the final predicted lesion.

In order to build the patient specific delay map, the gamma variate function of Eq. 1 was first fitted to the time-concentration curve of each voxel in the original perfusion image using Levenberg-Marquart algorithm. The delay was then estimated using the method of [19]. The resulting map is particularly noisy: voxels located in the edges of the brain surface, in the ventricles or in the heart of the lesion part lead to poor fitting results. In these areas, the contrast agent do not pass, which results in a very low signal to noise ratio and hence artefactual delay values. The performances of the fitting process was evaluated for each voxel using the sum of squared errors (SSE) after normalization of temporal signal height.

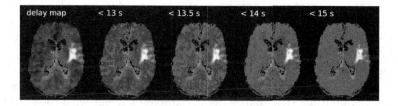

Fig. 3. Delay map computed for one slice of a patient with successive increasing thresholds of the delay. This representation gives information about the propagation of the contrast agent from the major arteries to the tissues.

Voxels with a SSE index superior to 0.20 were removed. The missing values were filled afterwards using an adaptative mean filter. Due to the anisotropy of perfusion images, this filter used was 2D. The optimal neighborhood size for every voxel was chosen so that at least 9 good fitted voxels were included. For visualization purpose, we used the wave front propagation representation proposed by [3] in Fig. 3. The resulting delay map was set as a new input of the simulator.

2.5   Evaluation of the Proposed Improvements

In order to evaluate the realism of the new version of the simulator, we predicted the final lesion of 8 real patients from associated simulated images using convolutional neural networks. A patient-specific learning approach was adopted: for each real tested patient, a model was trained only from its specific simulated

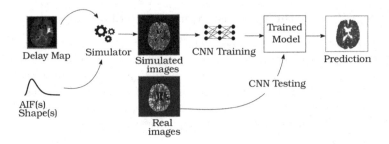

Fig. 4. General pipeline of the proposed approach.

images. We show the evolution of prediction performance, for different experiments, as we increase the degree of realism of the simulator. The general pipeline is shown in Figure 4.

Synthetic Training Databases. For each of the 8 patients, 4 different training databases were produced with an increasing degree of realism. In **database A**, the images were generated using a unique global AIF for all the simulations in the database and all the patients. The AIF parameters were set to the default settings of the simulator. In **database B**, a unique AIF was also used for all the simulations, but is different between patients. It was set according to the median signal of all the extracted specific AIFs for a given patient (see Fig. 2). In **database C**, a different AIF is used for every simulation. Each AIF was generated from the Delaunay representation of the extracted AIFs for a given patient, as described in Sect. 2.3. Finally, in **database D**, simulations were done using a set of multiple AIF shapes (as in database C), but with the additional inclusion of the delay map of the patient (see Sect. 2.4).

Network Classifier. We built a small neural network to provide a voxelwise prediction. The inputs of the network consisted in small 2D+t spatio-temporal patches of size (9,60) as described in [8]. These inputs were given to a pathway of two 2D convolutional layers: a first layer with 16 filters (size 2×2) and a second layer with 32 filters (size 2×2). This input pathway is followed by two fully connected layers: the first one with 15 filters and the second one with 2 output units as our task is a binary classification problem. Activation function in the hidden layer was ReLU and the one of the output unit was softmax. As long as the input patches have small dimensions and that convolution tends to reduce the output image dimension, we did not use any max-pooling approach to avoid further size reduction. We used dropout in the fully connected layers in order to avoid overfitting. We used the categorical cross-entropy function as a loss function and a stochastic gradient descent to optimize the model. All CNNs were trained using Keras 2.1.3 with Python 3.6.3 interface. The training of the networks took globally less than 15 min on a standard workstation with an NVIDIA GeForce GTX 1080 GPU with 8 GB memory (Fig. 5).

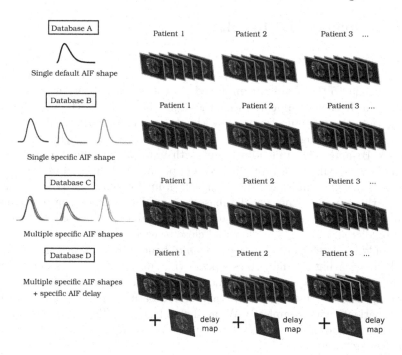

Fig. 5. The different databases considered in our experiments. Each corresponds to a different degree of realism that increases from database A to database D.

Experimental Details. A simulation is a volume of 25 slices, obtained by configuring the simulator with one or more AIF(s) and optionally with a delay map. Each training set consisted in 150 000 patches randomly drawn without replacement from 100 simulations (1 500 patches drawn per simulation). To ensured a balanced training dataset, half of the training patches corresponded to lesion voxels. The corresponding validation dataset consisted in 150 000 other simulated patches. For all training models, the total number of weights to train was 197 087, the dropout was set to 0.5, the number of epochs was set to 30, the batch size to 32, and the learning rate to 0.0001. Each model was trained 10 times and the best metric shot was given in the results. Each testing set consisted in all patches from one of the 8 real tested patients. For each database, 8 models were trained independently (a model per test patient). We assessed our results using the Dice and Hausdorff metrics. These metrics were computed between the predicted infarcted voxels and the mask of the final lesion provided by the follow-up FLAIR-MRI.

3   Experiments and Results

Dice and Hausdorff metrics associated with the lesion prediction ,from the 4 synthetic training databases are reported in Table 1. Each additional realism degree brought to the simulator improved the overall classification performance on real data. It clearly appeared that the adjustment of the AIF from the synthetic data to the real data is crucial: without any adjustment (database A), the average Dice is 0.15 against 0.39 after adjustment with one single specific AIF (database B) and 0.44 after adjustment with multiple specific AIFs (database C). The best classification performances are obtained with database D (*i.e.* by taking into account multiple AIFs and delays in the synthetic training data), although the improvement over database C is moderate. Note that database A has the lowest standard deviation among all databases: since all patients are poorly predicted, all scores are low and close to each other.

It should be noted that all patients seem to benefit from basic degrees of realism (like integrating specific AIF shapes), while only few patients benefit from finer detail improvements (such as modeling the vascular tree). In particular, integrating the delay into synthetic training database improves lesion prediction only for patients with complete CW, as shown in Fig. 6. These patients present alternative circulation in the vascular tree, and hence are more likely to see their lesion size regressing.

We can highlight that the best model so far from the ISLES ischemic lesion prediction challenge [21] presented an average Dice score of 0.31 ($\pm$0.24). Our prediction metrics are in same order of magnitude, even if we train only from simulated data. It is clear that these Dice score values are low. But prediction is a more complex problem than classical segmentation: a one-month delay separates the PWI-DSC input from the FLAIR ground truth, therefore all the predictive information contained in PWI-DSC are not always sufficient to precisely predict the final lesion.

Table 1. Dice and Hausdorff metrics between the predicted infarcted voxels and the ground truth final lesion. All the metrics are averaged over the testing dataset (average $\pm$ standard deviation).

Training database	Realism	Dice	Hausdorff
Database A	Single default AIF	0.15 ± 0.062	46.31 ± 2.9
Database B	Single specific AIF	0.39 ± 0.19	45.30 ± 2.5
Database C	Multiple specific AIF	0.44 ± 0.18	44.76 ± 2.5
Database D	Multiple specific AIF + delays	0.45 ± 0.18	44.66 ± 2.6

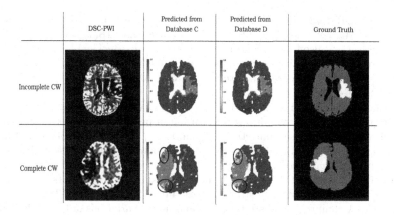

Fig. 6. Output predictions when training database C (2nd column) and database D (3rd column) for two test patients. DSC-PWI (1st column) is the real testing image. Columns 2 and 3 should be compared to the ground truth (4th column). Voxels in blue and red were predicted respectively healthy and infarcted. Patient in 1st line has an incomplete Circle of Willis (CW) while patient in 2nd line has a complete CW. Delay in database D seems to improve lesion prediction when CW is complete (see bold circles). (Color figure online)

4 Conclusion and Perspectives

In this paper, we demonstrated the possibility to evaluate a perfusion MRI simulator using convolutional neural networks for stroke lesion prediction. We trained several models on synthetic databases and measured there realism by testing the models on real patient data. Integrating increasing degrees of realism in the simulator improved the lesion prediction as measured by Dice and Hausdorff metrics. This realism was developed to model the vascular tree and benefit mostly patients with complete vascular trees. In this work, AIF and delay data were extracted from real patient images. In the future, we could have access to this data from computational fluid dynamics models of the vascular tree [22].

References

1. Calamante, F., Gadian, D.G., Connelly, A.: Quantification of bolus-tracking MRI: improved characterization of the tissue residue function using Tikhonov regularization. Magn. Reson. Med. **50**(6), 1237–1247 (2003)
2. Calamante, F., Yim, P.J., Cebral, J.R.: Estimation of bolus dispersion effects in perfusion MRI using image-based computational fluid dynamics. Neuroimage **19**(2), 341–353 (2003)
3. Christensen, S., et al.: Inferring origin of vascular supply from tracer arrival timing patterns using bolus tracking MRI. JMRI **27**(6), 1371–1381 (2008)
4. Davis, S., Fisher, M., Warach, S.: Magnetic Resonance Imaging in Stroke. Cambridge University Press, Cambridge (2003)

5. Frindel, C., Robini, M.C., Rousseau, D.: A 3-D spatio-temporal deconvolution approach for MR perfusion in the brain. Med. Image Anal. **18**(1), 144–160 (2014)
6. Georgiou, L., Wilson, D.J., Sharma, N., Perren, T.J., Buckley, D.L.: A functional form for a representative individual arterial input function measured from a population using high temporal resolution DCE MRI. Magn. Reson. Med. **81**(3), 1955–1963 (2019)
7. Giacalone, M., Frindel, C., Robini, M., Cervenansky, F., Grenier, E., Rousseau, D.: Robustness of spatio-temporal regularization in perfusion MRI deconvolution: an application to acute ischemic stroke. Magn. Reson. Med. **78**(5), 1981–1990 (2017)
8. Giacalone, M., et al.: Local spatio-temporal encoding of raw perfusion MRI for the prediction of final lesion in stroke. Med. Image Anal. **50**, 117–126 (2018)
9. Hermitte, L., et al.: Very low cerebral blood volume predicts parenchymal hematoma in acute ischemic stroke. Stroke **44**(8), 2318–2320 (2013)
10. Iqbal, S.: A comprehensive study of the anatomical variations of the circle of willis in adult human brains. J. Clin. Diagn. Res.: JCDR **7**(11), 2423 (2013)
11. Kellner, E., et al.: Arterial input function measurements for bolus tracking perfusion imaging in the brain. Magn. Reson. Med. **69**(3), 771–780 (2013)
12. Kudo, K., et al.: Accuracy and reliability assessment of CT and MR perfusion analysis software using a digital phantom. Radiology **267**(1), 201–211 (2013)
13. Livne, M., et al.: A PET-guided framework supports a multiple arterial input functions approach in DSC-MRI in acute stroke. JON **27**(5), 486–492 (2017)
14. Madsen, M.T.: A simplified formulation of the gamma variate function. Phys. Med. Biol. **37**(7), 1597 (1992)
15. Mahmood, F., Chen, R., Durr, N.J.: Unsupervised reverse domain adaptation for synthetic medical images via adversarial training. IEEE Trans. Med. Imaging **37**(12), 2572–2581 (2018)
16. Mukherjee, D., Jani, N.D., Narvid, J., Shadden, S.C.: The role of circle of willis anatomy variations in cardio-embolic stroke: a patient-specific simulation based study. Ann. Biomed. Eng. **46**(8), 1128–1145 (2018)
17. Østergaard, L., Weisskoff, R.M., Chesler, D.A., Gyldensted, C., Rosen, B.R.: High resolution measurement of cerebral blood flow using intravascular tracer bolus passages. Part I: mathematical approach and statistical analysis. Magn. Reson. Med. **36**(5), 715–725 (1996)
18. Pinto, A., et al.: Enhancing clinical MRI perfusion maps with data-driven maps of complementary nature for lesion outcome prediction. In: Frangi, A.F., Schnabel, J.A., Davatzikos, C., Alberola-López, C., Fichtinger, G. (eds.) MICCAI 2018. LNCS, vol. 11072, pp. 107–115. Springer, Cham (2018). https://doi.org/10.1007/978-3-030-00931-1_13
19. Rose, S.E., Janke, A.L., Griffin, M., Finnigan, S., Chalk, J.B.: Improved prediction of final infarct volume using bolus delay-corrected perfusion-weighted MRI: implications for the ischemic penumbra. Stroke **35**(11), 2466–2471 (2004)
20. Shin, H.-C., et al.: Medical image synthesis for data augmentation and anonymization using generative adversarial networks. In: Gooya, A., Goksel, O., Oguz, I., Burgos, N. (eds.) SASHIMI 2018. LNCS, vol. 11037, pp. 1–11. Springer, Cham (2018). https://doi.org/10.1007/978-3-030-00536-8_1
21. Winzeck, S., et al.: ISLES 2016 and 2017-benchmarking ischemic stroke lesion outcome prediction based on multispectral MRI. Front. Neurol. **9**, 679 (2018)
22. Zhong, L., Zhang, J.M., Su, B., Tan, R.S., Allen, J.C., Kassab, G.S.: Application of patient-specific computational fluid dynamics in coronary and intra-cardiac flow simulations: challenges and opportunities. Front. Physiol. **9**, 742 (2018)

Author Index